Hans G

Rolfing® Structural Integration for children and young people

Lebenshaus Verlag

Rolfing® Structural Integration
for children and young people

American edition, 2012

Published by
Lebenshaus Verlag
Schwimmbadstr. 46
79100 Freiburg
Germany

Translation into American
by Nicola Hanefeld

Printed by
Lightning® Source Inc., La Vergne, TN

ISBN 978-3-932803-13-0

Contents

Foreword

There are several books available on Structural Integration (SI), which is commonly known as Rolfing® *. However, no such book exists which deals specifically with the application of this method to children and young adults. The following book overcomes this information deficit and, as it is not widely known how valuable precisely this method is for young adults, is therefore especially useful.

My aim is not to simply inform readers of the possibilities and limitations of Structural Integration. I also wish to present a variety of suggestions to parents and educators of young people as to how they can offer support during and following the process of Structural Integration. In addition, I present information adding to the understanding of childhood development which is helpful for dealing with children in daily life.

Although superficially this book is „only" about *bodily* problems of movement and posture of young people, there is a lot of talk about psychological aspects as well as some anthropological considerations. This should not surprise parents because especially among young people the connection between the development of the body and the unfolding in soul and spirit cannot be separated. The book hence complements considerations on certain aspects of raising and educating children.

The founder of Waldorf Pedagogies, Rudolf Steiner, propagated the following maxim for bringing up children: „Conceive children in awe, bring them up with love, and let them go in freedom." It is not easy for parents and educators to live according to such a maxim. The media, science and economic factors „from without" appear to dominate and almost besiege children and families. These powers create trends in society setting parents and children under subtle, enticing or demanding pressure. It is hence not easy to find a way to incorporate flexible compromises whilst remaining true to oneself and being consistent without becoming closed to new insights.

In the section „helpful notes" details about books which deepen relevant topics may be found.

I would like to thank the many children and young adults whom I have accompanied along part of their life-journey. It has been my honour to see things through with you along the years.

Hans Georg Brecklinghaus

---

* Originally, the term „Rolfing" was just the nickname that many clients and practitioners gave this work. Then it became a registered service mark of the Rolf Institute® of Structural Integration in 27 countries.

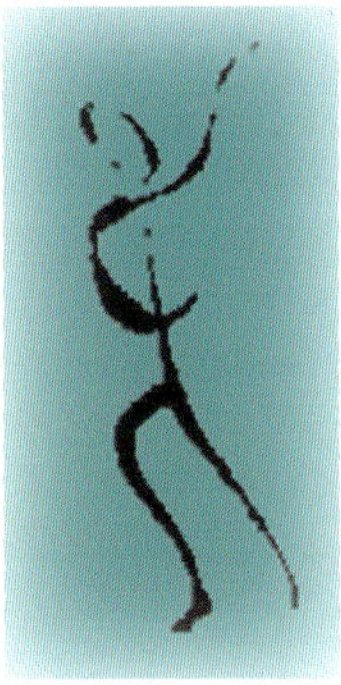

Introduction

When children suffer from backache or problems and limitations of movement, parents usually seek the help of orthopaedists who prescribe things like physiotherapy or insoles. Frequently, the results of such conventional methods are however, unsatisfactory.

The reason for this is that a local difficulty such as a spinal or knee problem cannot (or not alone) be locally resolved. Rather more helpful is a consideration of the static and patterns of movement of the person as a whole. Furthermore, an implicit shortcoming exists in trying to alleviate the named deficits only on a mechanical level. In the long run, a living organism is not to be repaired like a defective machine. Despite modern psycho-somatic medicine, conventional medicine usually ignores the fact that dealing with a person means dealing with a complex mind-body-soul unit.

Hence, one should not be surprised to observe that parents these days frequently seek holistic methods to help their children.

This book introduces *Structural Integration (SI)* which was developed by Dr. Ida Rolf. The most well known version of this method is Rolfing®, which is named after her. Structural Integration aims to improve body structure in such a way as to enable a person to unfold with less expenditure of energy and regain natural balance.

Dr. Ida Rolf (1896-1979) developed the method in over thirty years of work. While she was working as a biochemist at the Rockefeller University in the Twenties of the twentieth century she became especially interested in connective tissue. At the same time she became involved in Yoga, Homeopathy and Osteopathy. In the Forties she began working with people who had movement problems which could not be alleviated with conventional methods. Initially, she did this by teaching certain movement exercises that she had derived from Yoga. Step by step, she combined this with working manually on myofascial tissue (connective and muscle tissue). The decisive point being that she set the structure of the human body in relation to the higher level framework which gravity is.

Following application areas for Structural Integration may be mentioned: health care and prevention, reduction of chronic mal-tension, problems of body-static including posture problems, enhancement and optimising of movement, furthering body sensing and expression, reducing chronic mental-emotional tension, antenatal education, support during self-healing processes of chronic joint problems, etc.

An especially fruitful area of application is the work with children and young adults. Obviously, the above mentioned problems can be best resolved the earlier they are dealt with. Apart from this, adolescents react in a very natural way to the impulses that they receive during the process of Structural Integration which enormously supports this process.

The method is based on the following tried and tested basic assumptions:

1. Psychological and bodily well-being depends on a physique that is balanced and in a harmonious relationship to gravity. As most people are off balance, they are in war with gravity.
2. Our bodies can alter their gestalt and form during our lives. For this reason it is possible to subtly alter the relationship of parts of the body to one other by applying

a certain treatment to the connective tissue, and above all, to the fascia. This enables a more effortless inner alignment and ease of movement within the earth's gravity field.

3. During the process of Structural Integration a more aware body experiencing develops which can be understood as an altering expression of the person's being as a whole.
4. Inner alignment and a flexible and stable structure on the bodily side as well as psychologically are basic conditions for inner balance.

The above mentioned fundamentals are realised during Structural Integration on a practical level via a process which can be referred to in the broadest sense as a pedagogic one. So we are not dealing with a therapy defined in a narrow manner but of going down a path which activates the self-healing potential and healthy resources of a child. A learning process takes place on various levels: The organism learns via information from the nervous system and from the memory that living tissue has; the psyche learns with help of the organism; the spirit learns with help of the psyche.

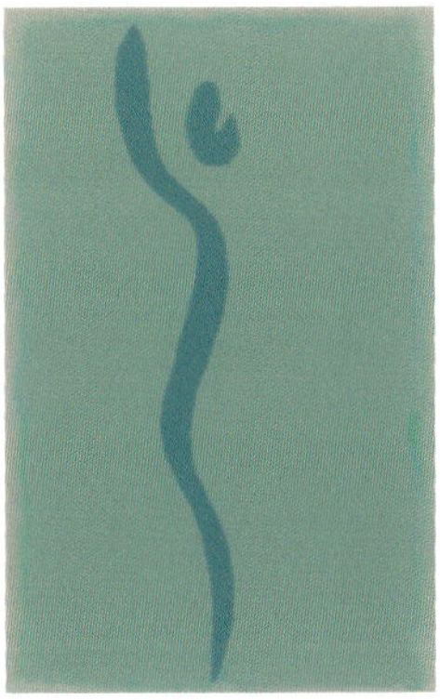

What Is Rolfing - Structural Integration?

1. Basics and Goals

Just like any other three-dimensional structure, the human body is subject to the influence of gravity. However, since gravity is energy that we neither see nor hear, smell nor touch, we are rarely aware of this simple but fundamental fact. Perhaps you know someone with one leg shorter than the other. If you take a closer look, you may be able to see that this person's spine has bent to one side in order to compensate for the uneven support. After all, the body's weight cannot be distributed evenly on uneven legs.

No matter what we are doing, whether we are moving, standing or sitting, we must adjust to gravity. In fact, we are constantly adjusting to it. Usually, we do this unconsciously with subtle changes of posture. We are never really still. Instead, we oscillate between slightly varying positions.

Adapting to the demands of gravity can be a more or less successful, more or less economical enterprise, depending upon the degree of balance we have attained in our body structures.

However: What do we mean when we talk about body structures of a Human Being?

The concept „structure" describes the mutual relationship between parts of a complex but unified entity. Structure deals with the principle organizing the parts of this unity. Since each physical entity is positioned in space, the concept of structure involves the three dimensions of space and therefore the relations between these dimensions.

The structure of each living being (including man)expresses itself as behaviour, for example in posture, movement and activity, but also in feelings, emotions, and in thinking. The diversity of posture and courses of movement in individuals is based on certain spatial patterns. These patterns form the structure of the individual, that is, the personal and specific form of someone's body. All physical beings or - we could say - their structure, are in constant interaction with the gravitational field of the earth. Therefore, if we discuss the structure of the human body, we mean not only the spatial relationship of the parts to one another, but also the relationship of the whole body - the whole structure - to gravity. Gravity affects our organism throughout life - it is a forming or deforming influence, according to how optimally or poorly a body is adapted to gravity.

The simple example of a pile of building blocks illustrates some of the major characteristics of structural stability: If the centers of gravity in all the blocks are precisely aligned on top of each other, the resulting structure will be stable and perfectly balanced. The organizational pattern of the structure, which is created by the spatial relations of the individual blocks (segments) with each other, is closely linked with gravity: A structure can only remain erect if its organizational pattern takes gravity into account.

Since the human body is also a three-dimensional structure in space, we can use the analogy of the block-model very effectively. In the human body, the individual segments would be: head, neck, shoulder girdle, chest, belly, pelvis, thighs, legs and feet (Fig.1b).

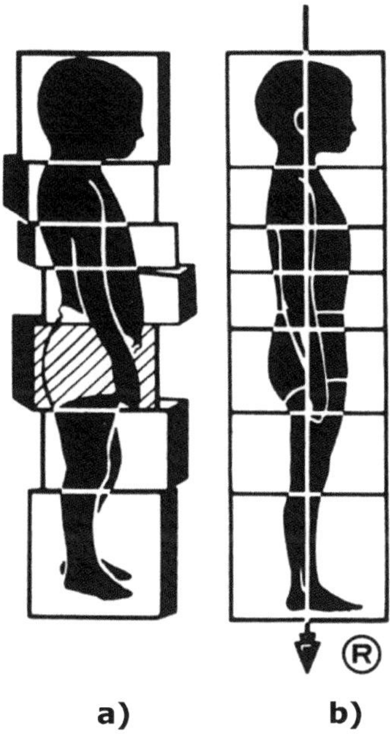

Fig. 1 Body structure of a standing boy

a) Unfavorable body structure with rotated and tilted segments

b) More economical body structure in relationship to gravity

If the segments of the body are well aligned, their centers of gravity all converge on an imaginary central line. If this line coincides with the axis of gravity, the weight of the body is transmitted vertically down to the ground and creates counterpressure upwards. This will support and uplift the individual segments (antigravitation factor). Thus, the organism needs to expend only comparatively little energy to keep itself upright.

You can easily check how well someone's particular structural organization promotes balance in the whole: If you look at their body from the side and imagine a vertical line through the middle, ideally, the following checkpoints should be very close to that line: ear, shoulder-joint, elbow, hip joint, knee and ankle. (Fig.1b).

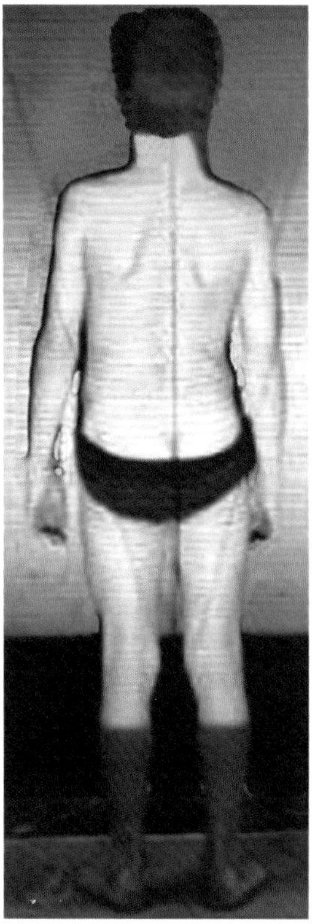

Fig. 2 Body segments are shifted horizontally to the sides and tilted sidewards.

If the segments of the human structure are, however, shifted (Fig.1a), their centers of gravity are taken away from the plumbline and the organism must expend energy to stay upright.

Segments can be shifted horizontally to the front, back or sides (see Fig. 1a and Fig. 2). Furthermore, they can be rotated around all or any of the three dimensional axes in space. Fig. 1a demonstrates rotations around the vertical axis. Moreover, the pelvis in this picture is tilted forward (rotation around the horizontal side-to-side axis).

Fig. 2 shows rotations around the horizontal front-to-back axis. The pelvis of the woman, for example, is higher on her right side than on her left side. This is compensated for by a opposite tilt of her shoulders.

A structure that is thus off balance must continuously fight gravity, which puts stress on the joints and tends to wear them out. Note also that the relative positions of all the segments are interrelated: the spatial situation of one segment will invariably affect all the others.

What determines the shape of the human body?

If you look at anatomy or physiology textbooks, you will find an elaborate version of something like this: The structure of the human „movement-apparatus" consists of the skeletal bones and muscles. The bones are the static element and provide support for the structure. They determine the basic shape of the human organism. The muscles are the motion element of the body. They cross the joints between the bones and contract to produce movement in the limbs. Descriptions of the fascial web are seldom included, despite the fact that the connective tissue actually constitutes the "organ of form".

Imagine for a moment that you could remove from your body all the intestines, organs, bones, muscles, in short, all the tissues except the connective tissue. What would you see if you looked in the mirror? You would see exactly the shape of your body, its contours down to even the slightest detail, in the form of a three-dimensional network of connective tissue.

All types of connective tissue - the superficial fascial „bodysuit", the fascial sheaths wrapping all the muscles

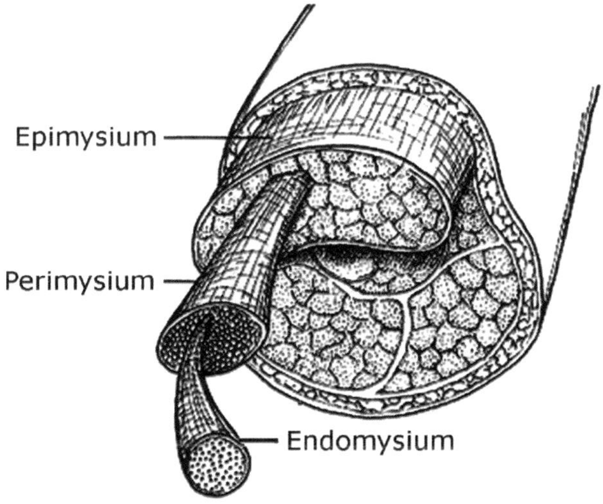

Fig. 3 Layers of fascia in a muscle

(fascia), the tendons, the ligaments, the fascial envelopes around organs, nerves, and blood vessels – do not only connect parts, as implied by the name. They also differentiate between various structures. In this way, connective tissue creates spaces in the body. The fascia of a muscle are wrapped around the muscle as a whole as well as its bundles and fibers (Fig.3).

The connective tissue, which surrounds and runs within and throughout the whole body, is a three dimensional and continuous network; it determines the positions of the bones and the body segments to one another by its respective state of tension. The fascia are also fundamental for the muscular balance in the body - the balanced tensional relationship between various muscles. For this reason Ida Rolf described the connective tissue as the „organ of structure".

Connective tissue has malleable qualities on the spatial and as well on the tensional level. This is, on the one hand, responsible for negative structural changes. On the other hand, the malleability of connective tissue can be used for positive processes of change.

The outermost connective tissue layer is called the superficial fascia. It wraps the entire body like one continuous body suit. Each individual muscle, as well as single muscle fibers and bundles of muscle fibers are wrapped in connective tissue bags. These bags are called fascia (Fig. 3) and are continuous with tendons and ligaments. In this way, the fascial system comprises a network of several superficial and deep layers. Since they all hang together, the fasciae allow tensional forces to be transmitted across several body-segments. The fascial wrappings of individual muscles determine how smoothly neighboring muscles can glide alongside or across each other. Moreover, the relative positions of the bones are determined by an intricate interplay of the various tensional forces of surrounding muscles and fasciae.

As mentioned before, traditional anatomy textbooks tend to focus too much on the skeleton as the fundamental static element that keeps the human body upright. I would like to contrast that image with another, which is equally exaggerated but describes functional reality better.

Let us picture the skeletal bones as being afloat in a mobile environment of muscles, tendons, fasciae, and enveloped organs. This environment of flexible tensional elements determines how, and in which directions, the bones can move. The bones only function as compressive elements in a tension-compression system. To make it simpler: you will immediately understand the image if you imagine a tent. Without the tent poles, the tent would of course collapse. It could not create any inside space. However, the position of the poles is determined and limited by the tensional pull of the fabric and ropes.

It is mainly gravity which is creating permanent tensions by pull and/or pressure in the body. Tensions by pull originate mostly in the fascial network, which is a closed system of bags in bags in bags. Tensions by pressure originate mostly in the parts of the body contained in the connective tissue membranes, i.e. in the bones and all other kinds of tissues being enveloped by connective tissue (hydrostatic model).

The key question of Structural Integration (SI) is: How must the parts of the body behave spatially to one another so that gravity has a positive ordering effect instead of a deforming influence on a person's structure, so that one can orientate oneself in gravity and straighten up effortlessly? (Fig.4)

The clearest criterion in finding an answer to this question is that of the economy of movement: Does the use of the body demonstrate a minimum of muscular effort during standing and whilst in movement? The more economic a person's movement patterns are, the more ideal the body structure is (and vice versa). It is then that apparently effortless movements are perceivable as graceful ones.

This approach not only leads to questions about the relationship between structure and movement, but also to questions about the relationship between structure and breathing, structure and metabolism etc. The relationship between body structure and soul also plays a major role. Posture is a mirror of the soul. Movements and gestures are always an answer of the soul to impulses coming from the inside or the outside.

What kind of influences can change a body structure?

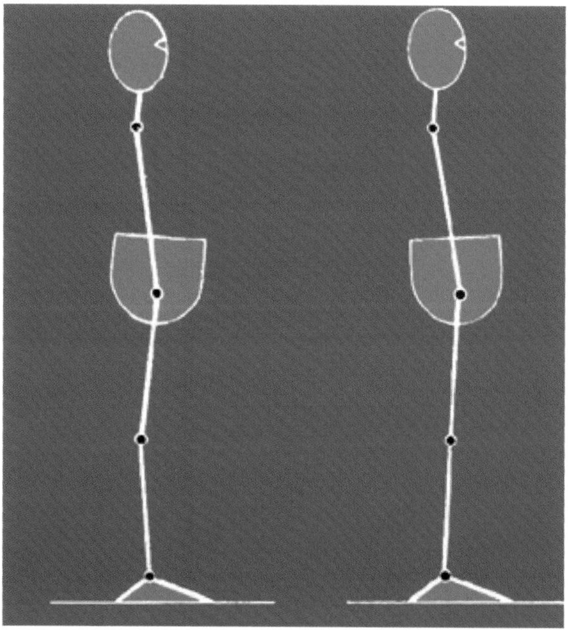

a) **b)**

Fig. 4 Two basic types of structural misalignments:

a) The pelvis is shifted forwards and tilted forwards-down, the knees are overstretched.

b) The pelvis is shifted forwards and tilted backwards-down.

When you observe people standing or walking, you will find that everybody moves differently; everybody has their own pattern of movement which is characteristic of them. However, most of us are not consciously aware of our movement pattern just as we are not normally aware of idiosyncratic behaviors. The various individual ways of holding ourselves upright and moving are first and foremost a product and an expression of our various individual life stories.

Let us start, though, with making a distinction between posture and structure. Posture, on the one hand, is voluntary; we can change and modify it whenever we choose. Structure, on the other hand, is not usually accessible to voluntary control. Therefore, it is completely useless to remind a child with a collapsed chest to „Stand up straight!" The child may be able to improve her posture for a few minutes. However, she will soon fall back into her usual slouch, because that is her structure - she cannot change her structure by simply making the effort. Habitual „good posture" does not come from holding oneself upright. It happens naturally when a body is free of structural limitations. The child is then able to stand upright easily and gracefully.

The experiences we make in a lifetime shape our body structures and affect how we move. Whatever life confronts us with emotionally or physically will leave an impact on our previous body structure. In this way, every new factor gets superimposed on the existing pattern and reacts with what is already there. Over time, elements of our personal history and environment blend with our reactions to them and form a complex, individual body structure.

Slight alterations in the static equilibrium of the body can over time develop into major structural flaws, with far-reaching effects on the available postural and movement possibilities. Emotional trauma, injury, invasive medical procedures, disease, and cultural habits (Fig.5) can result in structural fixations and a limited scope of movement patterns. Let's have look at two examples.

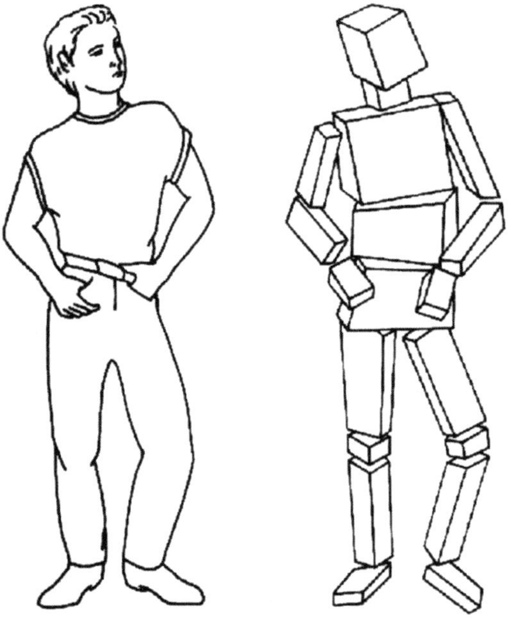

Fig. 5 Habitual posture

Susan suffers a sports injury to her right hip joint. Trying to give the painful side a break, she subsequently relies more on the left half of her body. The added strain causes the fasciae on the left side of the pelvis and the left leg to thicken and shorten; the muscles that are wrapped in them become less flexible. This produces uneven tensional forces within the tissues which further exaggerate the existing differences. Several segments of Susan's body are being pulled out of vertical alignment as her body tries to compensate for shortness in the left hip.

Joe has a hard time at school and at home. He learns that he has better be on his guard. For him, life means fighting for what he wants and needs.His posture reflects this: he is pushing his chest forward aggressively while retracting his shoulders. Although his posture is determined by an emotional rather than a physical condition, it will still manifest itself in his body structure as soon as the muscles around the thoracic spine and between the shoulder blades have become chronically tense. The myofasciae (muscles and their fasciae) of the upper back will shorten and thicken. Other parts of the body will structurally adapt. Joe may develop a swayback, for example, and overly straight knees.

Gravity will always tend to amplify those structural imbalances. Over time the structural patterns solidify.

But whatever the origins of structural imbalances, unfortunately the loss of structural order and economical motion is not the only problem: Tissues tend to form adhesions if they do not move properly. Wherever layers of tissue are glued together or thickened, the metabolism in the surrounding area will be impaired. Moreover, a chronically tense body will impede sensation as well as emotional flexibility. The autonomic nervous system will be recalibrated to match the constant tissue hypertension. Breathing will not be free and organ function will suffer. Just imagine what a permanently collapsed chest looks like and try to imitate that. Can you feel how difficult it is to breathe?

Moreover, a chronically tense body will impede sensation as well as emotional flexibility. The autonomic nervous system will be recalibrated to match the constant tissue hypertension. Breathing will not be free and organ function will suffer.

However, if - because of the plasticity of connective tissue - your body's structure can become less balanced and less stable, there must be a way to use connective tissue plasticity to bring about greater balance as well.

Biochemist Dr. Ida Rolf discovered just that. Her great accomplishment was to make a connection between body structure, gravity, connective tissue and body plasticity. In a lifetime of practical application, she developed an equally „simple" and brilliant method to balance body structures in gravity and allow them to align and uplift.

Goals of Structural Integration

When considering children and young people, we have to take into account that their current development is more to the fore than their personal history. Specific years of life have to be related to body-psyche developmental steps.

Despite the fact that Structural Integration (SI) can promote much more than mere physical change, a practitioner of SI is first and foremost concerned with body structure. The overall goal of Structural Integration is to reorganize body structure to move harmoniously with gravity.

This goal can be broken down to the following objectives:

1. Establishing the Line: Segments of the body should be organized around an imaginary inner line which in standing comes as close to the vertical plumbline as possible. This inner line starts at the top of the head and connects downwards in front of the spine, through the pelvic floor, between the knees and ankles to the ground. The line is a principle of organization for our bodies. All movements can start from the line and return to it.

2. Establishing optimum balance between front and back of the body (Fig.1, p.9) In trying to compensate for an unfavorable body structure, all too often people confuse overerect posture with upright alignment. (Fig.6).

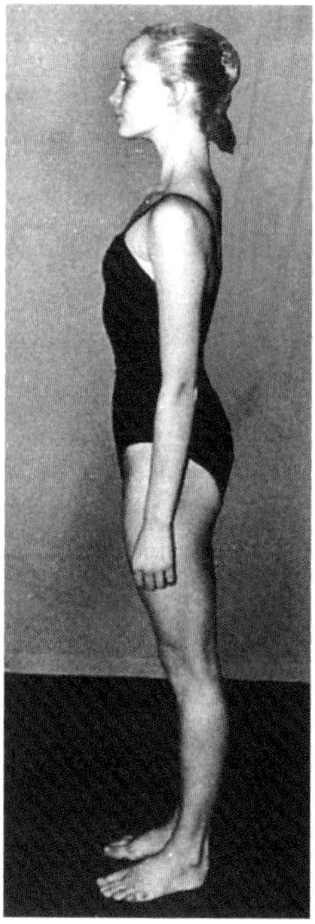

Fig. 6 Over-erect posture with a stiff neck, an upper spine being too flat and hyperextended knees

3. Approximating symmetry of left and right body-halves. This may include a certain amount of asymmetry since the left and the right side of the body are not the same inside: Most organs are not paired. Moreover, individual factors, such as left- or right-handedness, stand in the way of perfect symmetry.
4. The paired joints of left and right body-halves should be on a horizontal. If you draw lines through left and right ankle, knee, hip joint, wrist, elbow and shoulder, they should be in a horizontal plane parallel to the ground.
5. Balancing the tone of flexor and extensor muscles of the body (agonists and antagonists): Optimal economy of muscle effort is only possible if flexors and extensors cooperate instead of counteracting each other. When a flexor muscle contracts, the respective extensor muscle should be able to elongate freely. This is as true for the movement of individual limbs as it is for entire sections of the body - otherwise the body will have to shorten unnecessarily, and the core of the organism as well as the joints will be compressed.
6. Each movement should require the smallest possible amount of energy. In order to achieve this goal, movement impulses should not be obstructed anywhere. They should rather be able to reverberate throughout the entire structure so that the whole body participates in the movement, allowing it to be more flowing and graceful. Furthermore, upper body segments must be well supported from below.
7. To minimize the effort necessary for a particular movement, it should initiated with a reduction of tone in the antagonists and in the body at large. In the process of stretching the fascia of the muscles, the potential energy accumulated in the fascia can be converted into kinetic energy. Moreover, after this initiation, movement should be performed primarily by the deep, intrinsic muscles. The more superficial, extrinsic muscles should only kick in later. In this way, movement will start from the center of the body and translate into movement of

the arms and legs. The torso as well as the limbs will tend to elongate rather than shorten. We call this the extension mode of motion. Movement of this quality is always two-directional: it includes a settling down from the body center to where the overall motion starts (this is usually the direction of gravity) and the visible movement in the intended direction.

8. Freeing the breath will be achieved by creating enough inside space and sufficient mobility for the breathing structures to expand well.

9. Increasing sensitivity for the workings and sensations of your body as well as increasing awareness/mindfulness of what happens around you will open the spatial, emotional and interpersonal context for more harmonious movement.

Bear in mind that all these objectives are interrelated and that working on any one of them will help the others.

2. How We Go About Achieving the Goals

Generally speaking, we want to restore proper tension of the myofasciae, allow them to occupy enough space and have their layers and parts relate to each other well. This requires two things: differentiation and integration. Differentiation is the functional separation of body-parts and layers, which allows them to move freely and independently of each other. Integration, on the other hand, enables all the body-parts to cooperate and constitute a more complex entity on a higher level of organization. This will make the body move more efficiently and gracefully. Both aspects - differentiation and integration - are present in each Structural Integration session.

One way to achieve differentiation is by loosening and opening up adhesions. In a not so well-differentiated body, neighboring muscles are often „glued" together so that when we move, we have to engage muscles that are neither meant nor necessary for that particular movement. During a session, the practitioner releases these adhesions while the child/adolescent performs very specific movements. This will help him/her gain awareness and integrate a better movement pattern. It will also teach the nervous system that a specific movement is possible in a simpler, more effective way. In this way, the hands-on work and the educational aspects of Structural Integration complement each other to allow muscles to reclaim their appropriate space and proper functioning.

Differentiation also includes stretching chronically shortened fascia and muscles. However, the way we do it in Structural Integration, stretching is not a purely mechanical event. It, too, involves a learning process in the nervous system. Muscles and even more so their fascial envelopes have stretch receptors. They react to a slow but substantial stretching of the tissue by telling the central nervous system to permanently lengthen the fibers of the tissue. Therefore, manual stretching by the practitioner in

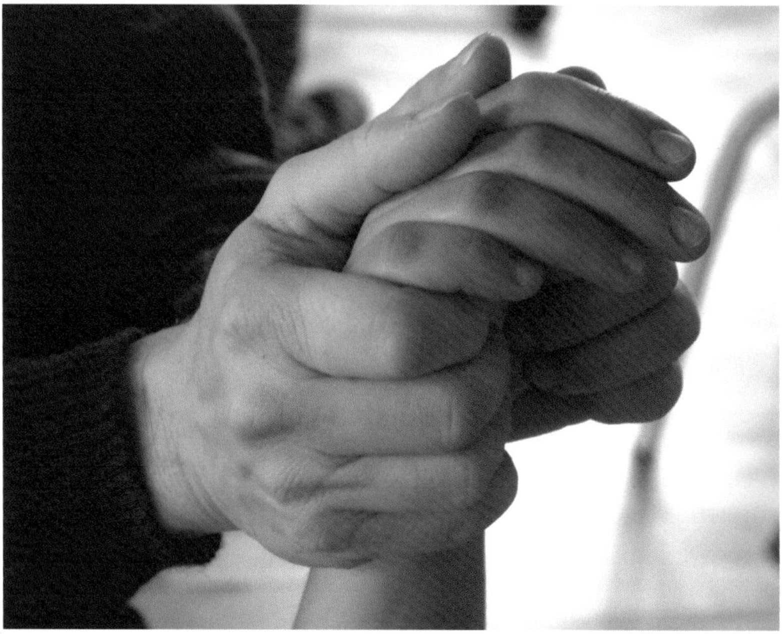

Fig. 7

combination with the client's active movement participation allows the body make lasting changes in the tensional relationships within its myofascial system.

The aspect of integration is most clearly present when the practitioner considers the internal connections and interrelations that are typical of a particular body-structure. He/she will do that anew in every single Structural Integration session. The work that is done in one area of the body not only changes that body-part, but also influences the way that part functions within the larger context of the whole organism. Therefore, by working one area, the practitioner may intend to achieve major effects in a completely different place. As it is so complex, integrating a structure is the far more difficult aspect of Structural Integration. To achieve true integration, it is essential to find a structural balance that caters to the various possibilities and needs of each individual client.

When we try to explain Structural Integration, we could also describe it as a predominantly nonverbal form of communication between practitioner and client. This communication develops on several different, yet connected levels and induces long-term change in the structure. One such level is neuromotor sensation. Structural Integration provides enhanced neuromotor feedback for your brain about what happens in your muscles and fasciae as you move. This feedback will help your nervous system give up old, ingrained movement habits and to develop instead new possibilities and better ways to move. It can also of course help rediscover lost possibilities. The connective tissue will be induced to continue reorganizing its spatial web after the series of sessions has been completed.

The second level of nonverbal communication has to do with somatic awareness. Structural Integration will help you become better aware of the wealth of sensations in your body. Feeling more, and more clearly, will encorage and enable you to be more sensitive to the positive and negative influences of your world on your body and soul. Moreover, the Structural Integration process will further a growing sense of the inner vertical line and the wonderful complexity of your organism. It can help you develop an intuitive „feel" for situations and an understanding of how you react and relate to your surroundings by adopting specific postures and movements.

The third level of nonverbal communication concerns the emotional realm. During a session, or in between sessions, emotional release may occur. People may laugh, cry, become angry or feel relieved. Moreover, physical as well as emotional trauma, which can be stored in tissues and in the autonomic nervous system, may surface during the process of Structural Integration. This can take the form of unconscious somatic reactions, conscious memory or new understanding. The practitioner will provide the space and support for the client to deal with such feelings and reactions. Rolfers do not normally provide talk-therapy like most psychotherapists, although in certain circum-

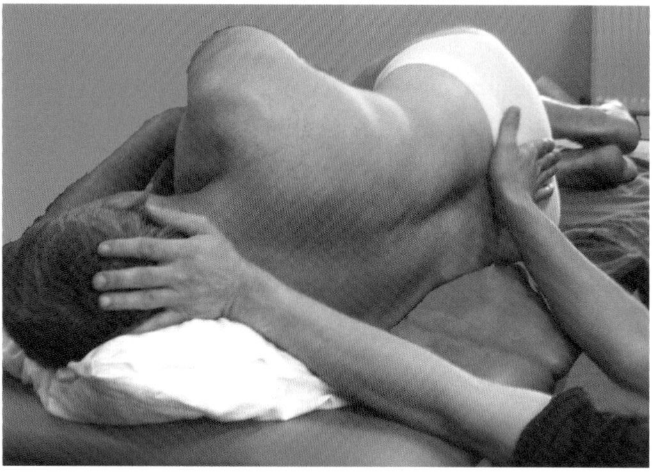

Fig. 8

stances talking may of course be helpful. Instead, Rolfers predominantly work on the level of the autonomic nervous system (Fig.8). When physical or emotional trauma is addressed in a session, the autonomic nervous system - simply speaking - starts a process of nervous system charge, in which the sympathetic branch is dominant. This is followed by a period of discharge, in which the parasympathetic branch takes over.

Rolfers have a wide array of techniques available to attain the goals of Structural Integration. The most prominent are of course myofascial techniques. Other techniques, such as craniosacral or visceral manipulation, have been taken from the osteopathic tradition. Various methods to develop sensory awareness and specific movement education are also included. (Fig.9).

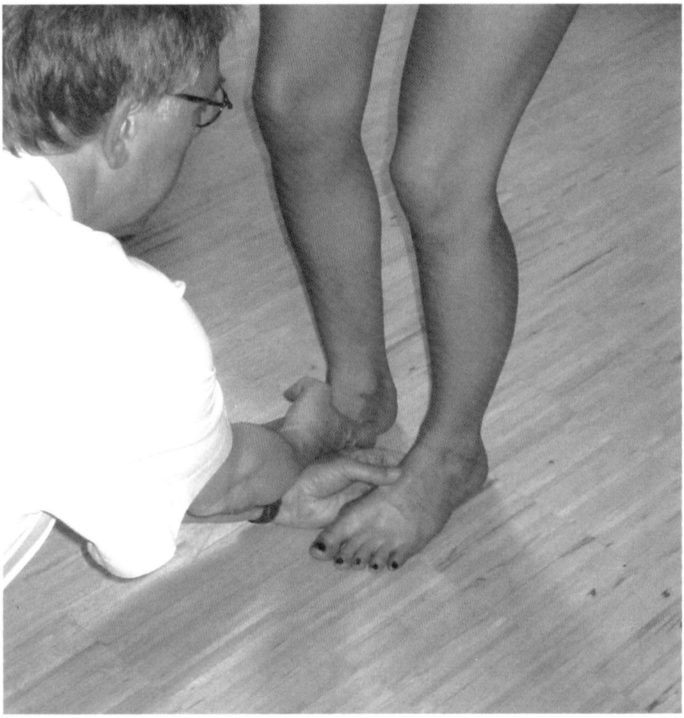

Fig. 9 Harmonic interplay of the joints of feet and knees in motion.

What happens in the process of Structural Integration?

The process of Structural Integration is a very personal one, because needs and priorities are individual. For example, while one child may tend to hold himself rigidly upright and therefore lack moblity, the other may be in a slouching position and have hypermobile joints. While one child may have high arches and a forward tilted pelvis, the next may have collapsed arches and a backward tilted pelvis. Some children may need greater stability and better grounding, while others will benefit from an increase in flexibility and lightness. Furthermore, structural problems may turn out to be of secondary importance in a session if psychological issues surface.

An initial interview provides you as parents and/or the adolescent with the opportunity to clarify needs and expectations.

The overall state of health will be talked over and you will be asked about illnesses or injuries. In general it is not opportune to discuss postural deficits etc. in the presence of the child. It is all too easy for the child to receive – albeit unintended – the message: I am not o.k. as I am. Therefore we as practitioners prefer to discuss these issues beforehand in the absence of the child.

Other topics might be the relationship of the child with parents, siblings, friends and teachers, the hobbies etc. This can give helpful hints for the process of Structural Integration. Sometimes we ask the child to paint the own body before and after the series of sessions. Thereby we learn how the child perceives its own body and in what way this perception might change over time.

Many Rolfers will take pictures of the young person from the front, back and sides before the first session and after he/she has completed the series. This will allow practitioner and client to see changes of structure. It will also help the practitioner prepare for the sessions.

Usually, the process of Structural Integration takes the form of a basic series of 10 sessions, with each session lasting – age-dependent - about 15-60 minutes. The intervals between the sessions vary between one week and several weeks. Longer intervals are sometimes reasonable, because we can follow up the development of the child/young person over a longer period. Often it is preferable or necessary to schedule one or more follow-up sessions per year, until the process of growth is finished.

The sessions with little children are playful, babies can be handled well while they are sleeping.

Because children are brought to Structural Integration by their parents, they do not come like adults with a will of its own. Therefore we take care that the child/adolescent has the option of saying "no" to the treatment. Often the response of the tissue speaks louder than words in determining whether the child/youngster wants Structural Integration or not (topically or basically). If the child directly or indirectly expresses that it does not want to come (anymore), we respect this and also advise the parents to do so as well. Maybe it is not the right time or there are other subtle reasons for this „decision" of the child.

On the other hand we experience over and over again that children feel „instinctively", that Structural Integration does them good. A wordless consent originates between the practitioner and the child.

If children – especially in the first sessions – like to have a parent present in the room, this is of course possible, although in some respects it is more advantageous – providing the child is of appropriate age – if parents are not present in the office. Experience shows that the expectations of the adults, or the relationship between children and parents more or less shape the behaviour of children/adolescents.

If the child - especially at the age of 3-7 years – does not like to remain lying down, this can be due to the fact that he/she evades problems and/or that he can badly focus or is hyperactive. In such cases it is helpful when a parent sits or lays down right beside the child and tells stories or reads to him/her.

A child sometimes does not tolerate a touch in a certain body area, e.g., on the head. This is due to the fact that the child feels that a problem exists right there. It is important that the practitioner respects such drawing of boundaries.

To promote the responsibility of children and adolescents and to do justice to her growing sense of self-determination, we encourage them to arrange appointments for potential post-ten sessions themselves (with cooperation of the parents).

In the time between the sessions the children experience not only structural and functional changes but also an altered relationship to themselves and to their environment. In the case of older children it is important sometimes to discuss these experiences and perceptions with them, so that they can be integrated into the personality and into daily life.

An optimal success of Structural Integration requires alert parental attendance in this time – an open-mindedness for new reactions and behaviour patterns of the child.

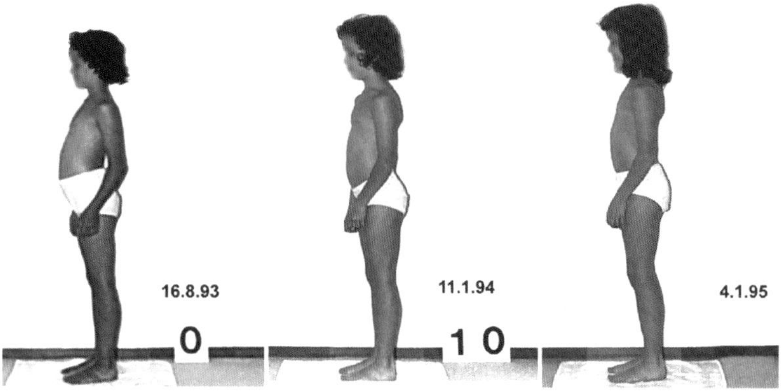

Fig. 10 Seven years old girl before Structural Integration, after ten sessions and one year later

How permanent are the results?

All living organisms strive for a higher level of organization and try to evolve a more refined complexity of their patterns. Add to that the fact that gravity reinforces indirectly body structures which are well-adapted to it and you have already two elements that will support permanency. Moreover, the balanced movement patterns that are developed in the process will enhance balance in the body structure. (Fig.10)

In addition, by the ensemble acting of tissues and nervous system, the organism will regain its capacity to self-regulate and release tension. For example, the child may experience a bout of hypertension in the neck and shoulder area and find after a couple of days that it has disappeared „all by itself". Before Structural Integration these tensions probably have been chronic ones. And experience shows that people who have been rolfed are better able to cope with physical as well as with emotionional stress.

However, the old saying „Use it or lose it" applies. The child will need to put its newfound sensitivity into action by honoring the body's signals when muscular tension or pain remind the young person to be more considerate and caring with himself. At this point you as parents are asked to support the child by serving as a model and by partnering your child in practicing exercises given by the practitioner.

Of course, life may confront anyone with a situation that throws them somewhat off balance again, such as severe illness, an accident or a psychological crisis. Supplemental sessions can help individuals cope and bring the system back to a harmonious balance.

How painful is Structural Integration?

Structural Integration is different for everyone. Some children feel only a welcome release in tension; others may experience quite intense sensations in some parts of their bodies as chronically tight tissues are starting to „melt". This can be described as a kind of pain, but it is most clearly linked with a sensation of relief and well-being.

Clinical pain research has shown that the sensation of pain is not a direct reaction to a sensory stimulus. Rather, any stimulus is transmitted across a large number of intermittent receptors and „interpretors" in nerves and the brain before we register pain, or in fact, any other sensation.In this way, stimuli are filtered and given significance by the peripheral and central nervous system. Life experiences play a big part in this process. Someone who has experienced a lot of pain in his/her life, may be predisposed toward that particular sensation and thus respond more quickly and strongly to intense stimuli.

Another child may have had to repress painful emotions such as sadness or despair repeatedly. When this happens, the emotions do not just go away. Instead, they are stored in the autonomic nervous system or held by chronic tension in parts of the body. In Structural Integration, such repressed emotions may surface in the form of physical pain. Of course, the body may also store memories of injuries or surgical interventions in tissues. Unconscious fear of change may also be transformed into painful sensations. So, the pain is usually not produced by Structural Integration. It only assists at times in bringing old pain to the surface, so that it can be addressed and ultimately resolved.

Remember, though: Whenever the child feels that disturbing or painful sensations are approaching his or her momentary personal limit, he/she can let the practitioner know by simply saying „Stop".

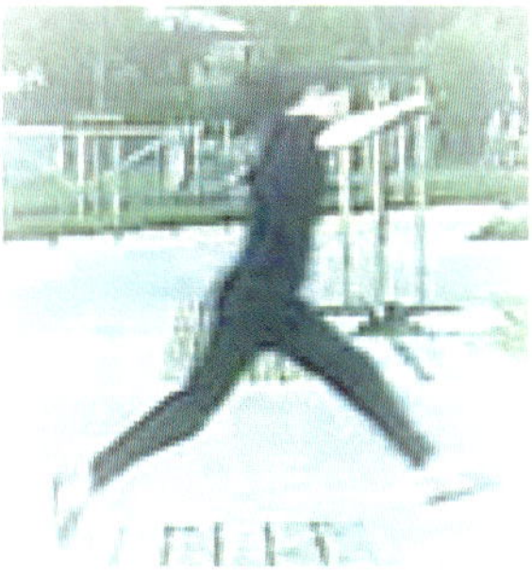

Areas of Application for Children and Young Adults

Parents who send their children for Structural Integration have roughly five different reasons for doing this:

1. The manifestation of a disturbance in the natural development of the child e.g. a mental or physical retardation.
2. The child is suffering from perceivable limitations of movement or posture, sometimes with pain.
3. Illnesses have been diagnosed that are not (or only partly) connected to the locomotor system e.g. asthma.
4. There are psychological problems which have manifested on the bodily level, e.g. chronic tension.
5. There is a wish to support the child who is involved in sporting or musical achievements.

These apparently very different issues are actually not so very far apart but overlap and complement each other. For the sake of clarity however, I would like to deal with each area separately in this chapter.

Having said that, here are some important considerations:

Structural Integration (SI) is not to be understood as a form of medical treatment. No diagnosis is made and no illnesses or symptoms treated. Parents whose children are not undertaking medical treatment are informed, if necessary, that medical treatment is pertinent or a necessary addition to SI sessions.

Generally, one can say that SI is equally suitable for the healthy as well as the unhealthy. It is implicit that symptoms which have their source in deficits of body structure, can improve. The initiation of this process is not however, via a narrow consideration of a single part of the body but rather a holistic consideration of the complete organism and the whole person. The aim is to create step by step a new order of the complete structure through which the person learns to deal more effectively with local problems (for example a rounded back). In this way, problems such as backache can become partially or totally superfluous.

Structural Integration (SI) is in some cases unsuitable or of only limited use. Cancer, strong spastic problems as well as brain damage belong to this category. Possible reasons for SI being unsuitable are clarified to the client by the practitioner prior to the first session. In cases which are not quite clear the relevant doctor has the last say.

Occasionally, parents wish to initiate changes in their child when it would be more appropriate that they initially (or at least in parallel) work on themselves. Children imitate their parents and use them as role models; they unconsciously mimic posture for example. Therefore it is an advantage when parents also experience the process of Structural Integration.

1. Age-specific Topics and Development

When considering children, we have to remember that their current development is more to the fore than their personal history.

During phases of growth, children or adolescents may experience pain in the periosteum (bone skin) or myofascial tissue. This arises when bones grow faster than the periosteum and the muscles and their fascia cannot adapt quickly enough. Consequently, the muscles have to compensate and may become hardened as a result. Manual treatment of the myofascial tissue can alleviate these growth pains.

Sometimes a child may display delayed bodily or psychological development. It has been repeatedly observed that a child overcomes such stagnation during Structural Integration. (Fig. 11)

Craniosacral treatment of the head can be helpful if a downright growth disturbance exists in the pituitary gland due to physiological reasons.

Reasons for growth disturbances sometimes lie in a prolonged medication with cortisone. Treating tissue with Structural Integration can sometime positively influence the flow of energy through it.

When we talk of the development of a person we naturally mean a holistic spirit-soul-body process. This is especially true for young people who are growing up.

In this context, a widely spread misunderstanding has to be corrected. Psycho-somatics should not be understood only as something *spatial* with the psyche affecting something in the body and the body affecting something in the psyche. It is appropriate to understand psycho-somatics also under *temporal* aspects. For the various parts of a human being's nature (physical body, life and formative forces, soul and the personal I) do not develop concur-

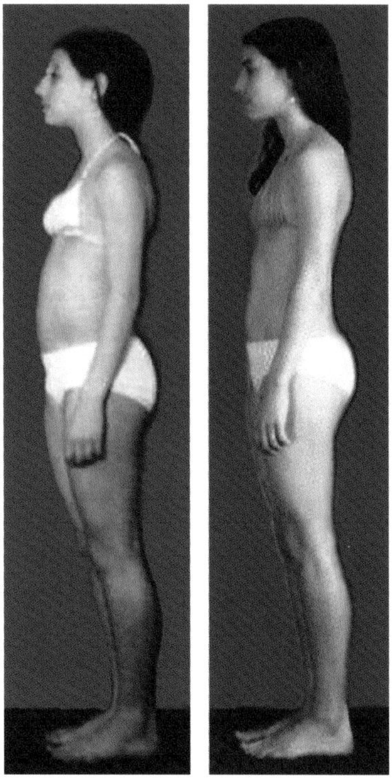

Fig. 11 A thirteen years old girl. On the left: still with a childlike hollow back. On the right: after three months and ten sessions of Structural Integration

rently but in different phases of life and in various manners.

Furthermore, the named parts of a human being have different functions and interact with one another in different phases of life in different ways. As we will see, this widened understanding of psycho-somatics will have very tangible practical consequences.

In the following paragraphs, the development of the young person will be divided into three seven year phases. Specific years of life will be related to clear body-psyche developmental steps.

This information on the developmental steps is anthropologically meaningful and justifiable. On the other hand though, there does exist the danger of understanding and applying them too schematically. It is not to be forgotten that each child has its own individual developmental process. Apart from this, there are transitions between the phases during which various abilities, of movement for example, can develop in parallel.

A third factor should also be considered. It appears that the development of children and adolescents, when compared with the first two thirds of the twentieth century is accelerating. This fact is due to two reasons. On the one hand, it appears to be an expression of development of mankind and is therefore natural. On the other hand, it appears to be the expression of a problematic erroneous trend in our culture that parents, therapists and teachers should be steering against even if, as in many cases, this is a challenge.

Children up to 7 years (the first seven year phase)

The parts of a human being's nature (physical body, life and developmental energies, soul and the „personal I") have different functions in different stages of life and interact with one another in various ways. For this reason when bringing up children one should only influence a certain part when this is „available".

The first seven years is primarily one of bodily development. This means that life energy during the first seven years is working on the development of the physical body. What is laid down as a constitution during these first years will effect the whole following life. That implies that the first seven years is decisive for later bodily and psychological health.

Life energy can only complete its work on the physical body if it is not misused for other things - for example, in the form of too early application of strong memory training and abstract intellectual learning. If this nevertheless happens, spindly growth may be the result as well as other physical and psychological consequences in the second half of life. Life energy lessens in the second half of life and is hence not as available to the body as it is then more active in the psychological-cognitive areas. Especially in the seven year phase between the 56th and 63rd (which is antipodal to the first seven years), one can observe adverse health issues if upbringing has not been optimally carried out. During this 8th seven year phase the events of the spirit and soul are not very related to the body.

For these reasons, parents should resist all attempts to allow kindergartens become „infant schools" and abuse these institutions as preparation for later schooling.

Early childhood ability to distinguish between various objects and animals and between different species and among toys with different patterns are sometimes taken as proof that children can think logically before they can even walk and speak. Sabina Pauen is a developmental psychologist from the University of Heidelberg: „Already by the age of seven months man is able to reflect on cause and effect."

This assessment is, however, based on a grave misunderstanding. When examining the „evidence" more closely that kindergarten children understand a great deal of Physics, one can see that the only safe conclusion is that children have an excellent perception, a good body feeling and an ability to store experience. Here one is observing body-knowledge and not intellectual knowledge.

Exactly in our times in which the psychological development of children is being threatened, we should tell them fairy tales. At best, from their third year onwards.

One reason for the loss of inner value systems is that parents no longer impart inner images via fairy tales or stories from the bible. Instead of doing this, one attempts to impart „social behaviour" intellectually or via moral appeals. Doing this is not only insufficient but also inadequate for this age group. „If we no longer tell children bible stories and fairy tales we'll land in barbarism." The Swiss philosopher Jeanne Hersch warned us in 1972.

A child lives totally in his or her perception of the world during it's first seven years. Influences come from without. Children learn through imitation. Especially the three basic forces in man – walking upright, speaking and thinking – develop from imitating.

The posture (Fig. 12) and moral attitudes of adults which children live with influence posture and moral behaviour of the child as an adult. Children witness what parents do and imitate it. This applies to the manner of dealing with non-living things but especially to living things (plants, animals and people.) This age group experiences social learning not from intellectual explanation or discussion but through what parents authentically live out in front of their children.

Typical childhood illnesses are not only useful for training the immune system of a person. They are also a confrontation of the crystallizing individuality with the „model" of the inherited body and hence forming the personal, individual body. It is for this reason that physiognomic changes occur that can be observed in children. Both aspects can be hindered through the undifferentiated application of vaccination and use of denatured baby food.

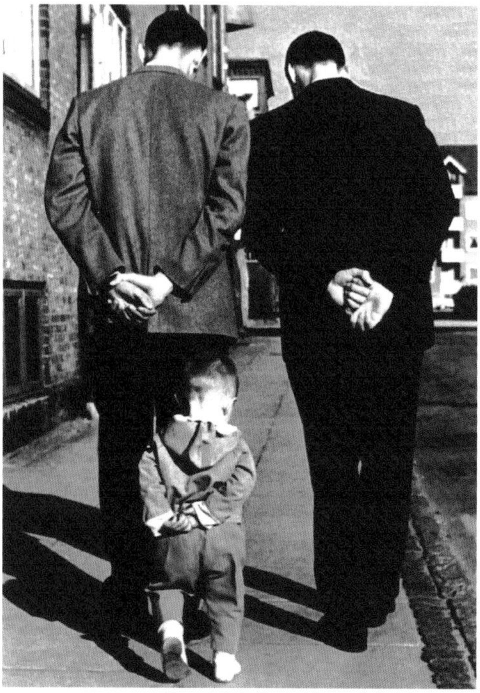

Fig. 12 Children learn from adults by imitation, including attitude, posture and movement patterns.

Babies and infants up to 3 years of age

Being born is the first great challenge that life on earth presents for man. Passing through the birth canal with bony parts (the sacrum and pubic bone), deforms the still soft parts of the baby's skull. After birth these parts usually move back to their normal shape and position. Sometimes, especially following a forceps delivery, they do not. Luckily, there is often a skilled midwife or doctor who can make the use of forceps unnecessary. Otherwise, a gentle manual correction from an experienced craniosacral practitioner can stimulate the natural self-regulation of the cranial bones.

Frequently the back of babies or infants is in tension because they have been pulled out too quickly during their birth. A light back massage can be helpful here.

A vacuum extraction can often be the cause of chronic headaches for the person born like this. I recall the case of 12 year old Pablo whose headaches only disappeared during Structural Integration.

A Caesarean is necessary in certain situations. Unfortunately, this operation is often carried out without being really necessary, with negative consequences for the child. The person misses out on experiencing the resistance of the birth canal. This may lead to movement problems at the crawling age and a difficulty in asserting oneself in later life. A certain compensation for this can be therapeutically initiated if a practitioner repeatedly holds the feet of the new born baby while at the same time holding the upper back. One must also critically comment the use of artificial hormones during labour because they disturb the natural course of a birth. This can result in a life long disturbance to the vegetative nervous system.

Premature babies often suffer from colic attacks, migraines or asthma. A structural or vegetative treatment can ease these effects or relieve them completely.

Around the age of 2 1/3, during the 3rd year of life, when the nervous and sensory systems have developed, the child begins referring to itself in the I-form for the first time. One can speak here of the first birth of the „personal I." From the moment of the first personal-I experience the child is able to remember. This means that it develops the sensation of being a continual instance within altering experiencing. Individual self awareness begins to develop – for „I" and the world are no longer one. This self-awareness attempts to affirm itself during the defiant phase.

How does the child develop during these first three years? When we say that a child grows, we associate automatically the idea of growth from below upwards. Actually, an embryo develops from the head downwards.

Certain structural characteristics that in later years may need treatment are normal for an infant and should therefore not be a cause for concern.

Bow legs are, for example, up to an age of 2,5 years normal because bone growth on the inside of the knees until this average age occurs faster than on the outer side of the knees. Rickets (vitamin D deficiency) or inner resistance to development can have a retarding effect.

Furthermore, a dominating C-curve of the spine is the normal shape in babies. When a child learns to walk, up to an average age of about 7 years, a hollow back develops associated with a forward and down tilt of the pelvis.

During the crawling phase, this develops because the back muscles develop more rapidly that the ventral muscles. Hence the two Iliopsoas muscles are used as soon as the child can walk pulling the lumbar region into a hollow back and creating the pelvic tilt.

If these structural symptoms are still observable into the eighth year of life, a corrective structural treatment is recommended.

Small children often have a tense neck because the head is big and heavy in relation to the rest of the body.

Learning movement and walking takes place in the following order. The mentioned stages are average ages. Premature babies go through the stages approximately 1 – 2 months later.

Ability	**Age**
Turning to the side	with 18 weeks
Turning onto the stomach	25 weeks
Movement biased as the sides of the brain are not yet fully connected	first 4 months
Supporting itself upon the lower arms and lifting head	4-5 months
Landau-Reflex; lifting the head, stretching spine and legs whilst „swimming" while lying on the front.	6 months
Turning from front to back	30 weeks
Supported by the hands lying on the front, head turning.	5-7 months
Crawling whilst sprawling on front side	40 weeks
Crawling on knees and hands	46 weeks
sitting	11 months
standing	1 year
walking	1,5 - 2 years

I would also like to add that a sideways curved position with a head turned to one side is normal during the first few weeks of life.

If you are not sure that your child is developing normally consult your paediatrician who is generally more informed about early child development than an orthopaedic specialist.

Infants are not minature adults. We have already observed this with respect to the typical body structure (hollow back development) and the initially developing motor abilities. In addition, the body's centre of gravity lies higher in children than in adults – approximately at the 12th thoracic vertebrae. In adults it lies at the height of the third lumbar vertebra. One should also note that the connective tissue of babies consists of about 80% elastic fibres – the number of collagen fibres is still small. The connective tissue is adapted more to movement than stability at this stage. The quality of connective tissue that an adult has is reached around the age of 12 – 14 years of age. Babies also have areas of cartilage that are not yet bony and therefore still malleable, for example the back half of the foot, parts of the pelvis and the cranial bones. All theses differences between adults and children make a careful treatment which is adapted to the child a necessity combining a cautious handling considering all the child-specific conditions which are present.

It repeatedly happens that parents force the development of movement in their offspring. The reasons for this are manifold. Some fear that their child is developing too slowly. Others interfere due to ambitiousness „my child can already ..." The tragedy being that they are harming the development of their child. In Structural Integration we are time and again confronted with the consequences.

For this reason the following appeal to you as a parent: Respect the natural individual rhythm of movement development of your child. The child has to gain new abilities *on its own* and *in its own time*.

Do not entice the child to do certain things and do not help him or her to do them. Otherwise the development of the abdomen and back muscles may be hindered. Vital nerve circuits cannot develop and space for the evolvement of the brain stem is limited. The later is responsible for proprioception and contending with gravity. As a result movement (also at later stages) becomes controlled more from the cerebrum and the „interbrain". Movement becomes inefficient and the cerebrum and „interbrain" are not free for performing their real tasks. Making up for developmental stages that have been missed out is difficult as children, once urged to move to a next stage, do not wish to go backwards.

So do not sit your child up if it cannot sit itself up. Too early sitting in this context can be the cause of a rounded back (kyphosis) and of a too flat thoracic spine. Only use carrying devices that give the back a firm support so long the child cannot sit on its own.

It is not good to stand a child up that cannot yet stand on its own. One should also avoid the popular game where the child is lifted and animated to push up with its legs from the adults thighs. At this age it is only a stretching reflex and not yet a standing-up impulse. And last but not least, if the infant cannot yet walk without help, do not take it by the hand so that it can take its first steps.

All this supposed help leads to neuro-physio-logical disturbances, in later years maybe spinal damage, flat feet etc. because the bones, muscles and neural circuits of the child are not yet sufficiently developed.

What you can do and what you should do: Make sure the infant has enough space to move, clothes allowing for movement and a not too soft surface where the child lies. A child needs a free selection of toys and above all attentive interest and empathy during it's efforts to learn new things.

When a child becomes frustrated from leaning from trial and error and is in tears or is angry feel with your child but do not „help" it. (Dangerous situations are here obviously excluded.) When a baby cannot free itself on its own out of an unexpected situation and starts to cry, put it back to the original position or just free it from the awkward position.

Here further advice for your everyday life with a little one:

- Carry a baby in *lying* position and support the head and body when propping it (eg. for winding). When lifting a baby out of bed keep it in the *lying* position whilst supporting the buttocks, shoulders and head.
- If you have taken a crying child into your arms do not put it down until the baby has noticeably relaxed visible for example by an involuntarily deep inhalation.
- The prone position which is often traditionally recommended for babies is not conducive to movement development; it is even detrimental for it. Neck muscles can cramp in this position.
- Sleeping on the abdomen with crossed over feet can lead to pigeon toes (talipes varus) and is also associated with a higher frequency of SID (sudden infant death).
- Bodily contact is one of the most important things that you can give your child. Not the essential but a hardly considered reason is as follows: An infant that has experienced little bodily contact will experience tender body contact later, when sexuality awakens, in certain circumstances as unpleasant or embarrassing being only associated with sexuality because it has never experienced non-sexual body contact.
- The penis of male babies should only be touched gently otherwise the tissue around the penis may tense and shorten. This, in turn, may influence the tension relationship of the pelvic floor and legs which may bring structural deformities to the fore. When you wash the penis do not pull back the foreskin until it is loose enough to move back without force. Otherwise it may tear and troublesome scar tissue may be the result.

Children from 3 – 7 years of age

The impulse to ask „why?" develops in the 5th year of life. The child starts trying to extend its´ consciousness towards life and into the world. It is tempting for adults to answer these questions on the cognitive level with adult knowledge and the use of simple words. More service is done to a child however, if one answers in pictures, images and stories.

Sending a child to school too early at the age of 6 or even 5 has a disadvantage in later life, above all in the 7th seven-year phase between 56 and 63 years of age. A Swedish saying says „bright children often make for old fools." The reason for this being that life energy is taken too early from the physical body through a too early activation of the power of memory. The bodily deficit relating to age-based physiological development of the nervous system then becomes evident in old age when normal bodily degeneration sets in.

It may happen that due to its development a child between four and six years of age stutters for a while.

With regard to structural and functional development, one must consider again that a premature baby has a normal delay in development of 1-2 months.

The normal combination of a forward and down tilted pelvis in children up to the age of 7 years has already been considered. This is frequently associated with a slight over-stretching of the knees.

Slight knock-knees are normal between the ages of 2,5 – 8 years because in this age bone growth occurs faster on the outside of the knees than on the inside.

Up to the age of 4-5 years of age it is normal for the arch of the foot to be flat because ossification is not yet complete. If you are not sure whether flat feet (associated with heels pointing outwards) might be a malformation that should be treated with Structural Integration you can perform two tests:

Whilst standing, get your child to lift its big toe. Now get the child to walk on its toes. If in both cases an arch of the foot forms and the heel no longer points outwards you need not worry. Otherwise, Structural Integration can be helpful in assisting the development of a functional foot arch. (See page 68 f)

Following abilities belong to normal functional development: A child can stand on one leg at the age of 4 and can run by the age of 5.

Initially, in small children, the deep inner body muscles are more developed than the superficial muscles. This means that children are compact on the inside but soft on the outside because they do not yet have their structure „under control". Later on they use the outer muscle layers more until maturity and the inner muscles less as the inner muscles are not as strong as an adult musculature.

Problems that need treatment like a weakness of the connective tissue in outer tissue layers, flat feet with heels pointing outwards (splay-foot), scoliosis and a round back often show up around five years of age.

A common way of sitting in our culture is kneeing down between the feet with the thighs to the inside and the lowerlegs plus feet turned outwards. This position can result in a structural inward rotation of the femur and pigeon toes.

Before we consider the second 7 year phase, I would like to point out an interesting phenomenon. Small children have a way of bending that is advantageous for the back and from which we could learn. They bend from the hips and not from the back and push their buttocks back to compensate the weight coming from the upper body which tilts forward. Balance is hence optimal and the torso remains elongated. (Fig.13).

This way of moving is however usually lost between the ages of three and seven years of age as the children imitate and orientate themselves upon the example of their mother or father. These role models are everything apart from exemplary as most adults bend downwards out of their back. Even if they at least bend their knees while they bend, they usually round their back and the whole torso is compressed to the fore. Such uneconomic and joint burdening ways of moving are the basis for structural difficulties that develop later with symptoms such as backache, painful joints between the pelvis and sacrum, lumbago etc..

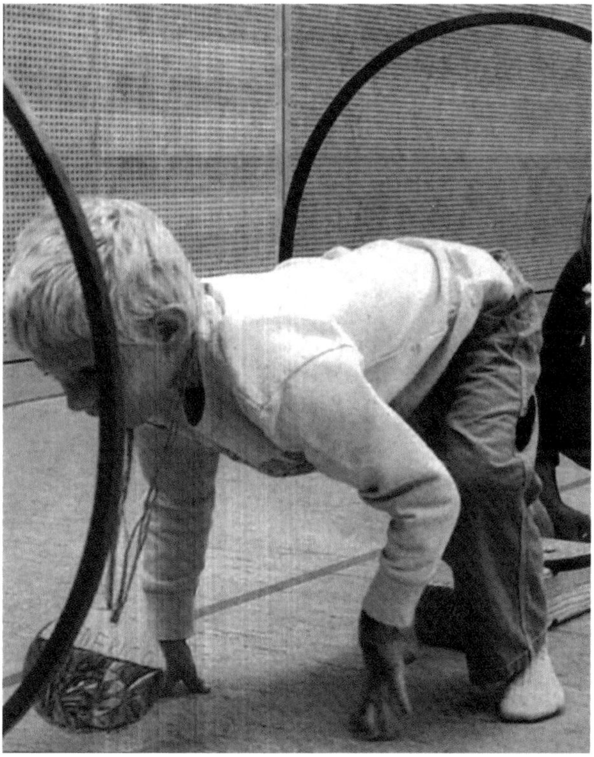

Fig. 13

Children between the ages of 7 to 14 years (the second seven year phase)

Aptitudes, habits, character, learning abilities and fantasy develop in the second seven year phase. The mind and psyche of the child are predominantly busy with the development of these life developmental processes. For this reason we should only *indirectly* influence the mind and psyche of the child. Fairy tales and stories, images and parables, memory training and guided fantasy are media with which to best support this process.

The child develops individual feelings during this phase (second birth of the personal-I). It may be sometimes withdrawn and dreamy but in certain situations also aggressive towards parents and teachers. The distinction between good and bad and between ugly and beautiful develops. We can increasingly speak of the child's personal conscience and own power of judgement.

There is a lively exchange from within to without and from without to within; of giving and taking. The child learns now less via imitation but more from reverence and love of the people it experiences as a true authority. A balanced relationship between authority (boundaries) and love is necessary so that the child becomes neither extroverted nor introverted.

Especially norm-internalisation and habits develop during this seven year phase. Daily and yearly regulated routine is important so that no problems with sleep, digestion, heart rhythm, asthma, polyarthritis or other rheumatic illnesses develop.

Between the ages of 7 – 14 any illnesses are caused less from within (as during the first 7 year phase) rather more from without, the environment. For this reason children between the ages of 8 – 14 are potentially least threatened by illness. Sources of illness and disease are poor quality of food, too many intellectual duties and responsibilities with too much stimulation of the child's naïve power of judgement as well as limited or stereotype movement.

At the age of about 14 children become sexually mature. However, it is to be observed that girls reach maturity earlier these days. Research from Florence and the United States indicate that excessive television consumption by young people may be responsible for this due to the production of lower levels of melatonin. Low levels of melatonin play an important role by early puberty. (*Spiegel Online*, June 29, 2004)

Balance problems between the ages of 7 and 8 as well as between 12 and 13 are often normal and pass. The reason for this is that the arms and legs grow faster than the rest of the body. This is also the cause of the occasional gawkiness that can be observed at this age.

In contrast we should not overlook the fact that problems with overweight in the generation that is at present growing up is a serious problem. Many school children do not have enough movement in everyday life and nourish themselves poorly.

The increase in movement and motor disturbances is alarming. Too many children have deficits in their motor-sensory coordination ability. Many of them are unable to balance on a bar or cannot even walk backwards. The rise in accidents in primary schools is linked to poor coordination abilities. Experience shows that Structural Integration is a possibility to compensate this deficit.

However, the onus is on parents and school to change the life and learning circumstances of children. Children sit long hours in the classroom, whilst doing homework and in front of the television. In the past, little tasks like going out to fetch a friend, carrying a bag of potatoes or bringing empty bottles to the milkman were taken for granted. Today we have to deal with a loss of „childhood on the streets".

Many factors have contributed to this situation: Urbanisation and traffic has led to cramped and dangerous living

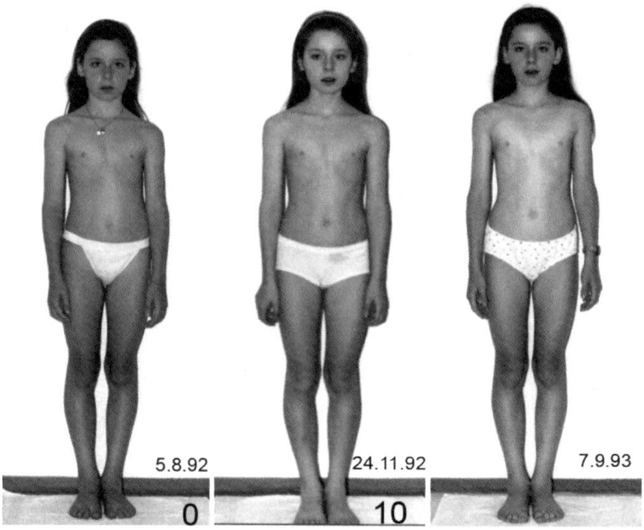

Fig. 14 A 10 years old girl before and after ten sessions of SI and nine months later

space. Many parents have the habit of taking their son or daughter somewhere by car instead of sending them on foot or by bike. In addition, there are long phases of sitting at school without adequate breaks for movement and long periods in front of the computer or television.

There is evidence that children who have experienced Structural Integration rediscover their pleasure of movement. This supports their success with learning as all cognitive accomplishment begins with motion.

Children discover their world with their bodies and hence become aware of themselves using their arms, legs and hands for orientation. Only when a child experiences its´ body does it develop a sense for its´ abilities and limits. The child who gets away without a scar on his knee will never experience how fast one can go around a corner on a bike.

Some children have learning difficulties because they cannot easily change from using one side of the brain to the other. Here, subtle work on the cranial bones can improve the flow of cerebrospinal-fluid.

Between the ages of seven and the start of puberty are often the best for Structural Integration. The children are open, cooperate well and have an enormous potential for change. (Fig. 14.) It is recommended to treat children older than 11 years of age alone as they engage better when parents are absent.

Adolescence (third seven year phase)

The inner emotional world is fully formed by the age of 14. The musculature and sexual organs now increasingly develop. The person takes a step towards consciously encountering the outer world with his or her metabolism, locomotion and sexuality which culminates at the age of approximately 19 in a sort of third personal-I birth. Career wishes and choice usually fall within this seven year phase.

Young people experience an inner tension between the awakening of sexual urges and high ideals within the realm of reflection, emotion and will.

Consciously redirecting from within to without can lead to rebellion against dishonesty and unfairness. This rebellion either has its´ emphasis on the cognitive level, (philosophising, brooding over things) more often in the emotional area (music, literature, drugs) or most frequently in getting one's own way (destructive behaviour or wanting to change the world.)

Step by step parents should let and set the young person free. It is not easy to find a balance between setting boundaries and trusting. On the one hand boundaries can strengthen the personal-I of the young person, on the other hand becoming self-responsible can be learnt when trust is offered and space given. A respectful dialogue should increasingly replace parents' power and friendship should replace authority.

Young adolescents are sometimes not motivated to come to Structural Integration. As parents have often taken the initiative it may happen that the young person projects tension and rejection towards the practitioner. It may happen that a girl sabotages working together with the practitioner to „prove" to her parents that there is nothing that can help her chronic backache.

If an adolescent does come, the practitioner must respect that this phase of life involves major biochemical

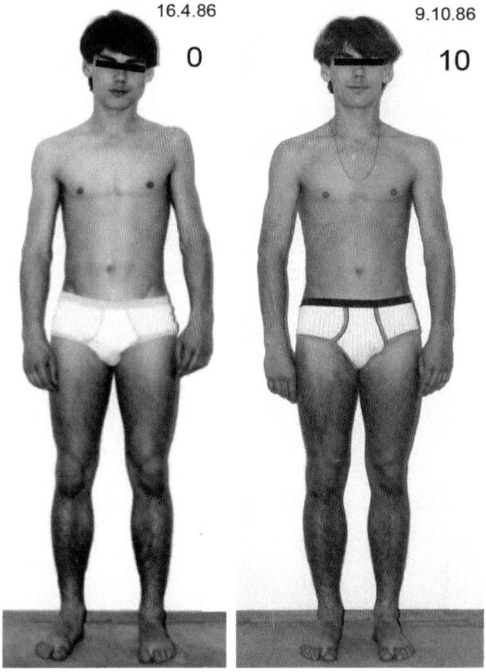

Fig. 15 An 18 year old adolescent before and after ten sessions.

and psychological change. In extreme cases, treatment may be just too much.

The posture of a young person can often mirror inner conflict. Additionally, we should not forget that young people often need an exaggerated „cool" or extravagant posture (and movement patterns) to protect their self. For this reason it is helpful for Structural Integration initially to work towards mobility, permeability and stability of movement and then towards good posture as expression of good structure.

It is of importance that the practitioner conveys his of her personal standpoint openly and honestly so that unpleasant or critical situations are not swept under the carpet.

2. Posture and Movement Problems

Wide general opinion says that inheritance plays a role in certain posture or movement problems („It is in the family."). One now knows however, that genes do not truly have the last word in this area. Structural problems, imitation and / or social embedment with a certain psychological climate may have been influential factors. This does not mean that certain constitutionally set limits should not be considered.

Obviously, structural problems have a better prognosis when they are dealt earlier rather than later in life. This fact makes Structural Integration so valuable for children.

I would like to clarify this aspect whilst considering various postural deficits and movement problems.

Chronic tension

Chronic tension is a classic area application for Structural Integration. For example: chronic shoulder and neck tension. The cause of shoulder and neck tension is almost always to be found directly or indirectly in the structure of the whole body. It is for this reason that massage that only treats the shoulder and neck regions rarely is of lasting success. Frequently one can observe that the underlying regions are not adequately supporting the neck and shoulder areas. This leads to overstrain of the muscles in this part which are trying to keep the head upright. An example of this being a sunken chest which pulls shoulders and neck forwards. When this happens, the shoulder girdle and head are no longer vertically aligned over each other but are positioned *in front* of the body's gravity axis. Naturally, the shoulder and neck muscles then progressively shorten or harden. A collapsed chest is in turn held in position by short and tense stomach muscles.

The jaw musculature

A key chronic high-tension area in the body is the jaw and associated muscles. Neck tension and headaches can come from teeth grinding at night. Pain from the muscles involved in chewing can also spread to neck areas and cause headaches. Dentists call this phenomenon bruxismus which is premature and unnatural erosion of the teeth involving abnormal biting patterns.

Obviously, the aim of Structural Integration is not to just relax tense muscles, in this case the mastication muscles. This applies to all tension problems. The successful approach should consider all varying factors. One aspect is the relationship of the lower jaw to the skull and cervical spine. A second aspect being that movement patterns and the tension state of the tissue of both jaw joints can vary. A further difficulty to consider is as follows: Mastication muscles that have long been cramped and perhaps painful have created a kind of high tension which in turn hardens and affects the muscle tonus in general. This vicious circle can only be alleviated and regulated step by step.

Here I would like to mention something that has become more and more frequent in recent years: The use of braces for supposed and real tooth and jaw malalignment. Nearly 50% of all young people today wear a brace. Sometimes it is almost a status symbol or a type of style accessory. He/she who has one is „cool".

However, these trends have not been created by the children and adolescents. It is the lobbyists from the health care branch who propagate treatment of the dentition with a brace. The costs are not to be underestimated.

Recent studies make one think: Positive results seen over the longer term of thirty years lie only by 20%.

Much more serious is however, that braces which fix both upper jaw bones with each other (Fig. 16) hinder the subtle mobility of these bones which frequently results in vegatative dysfuction and cause headaches or migrane.

Fixed braces can also worsen an existing scoliosis. A long-term consequence can be dysfunction in the jaw area caused by treatment with braces. The dentition is additionally an essential part of the fine regulation of mastication and neck muscles. It also has an orientational function for the growth of the facial skull. From the viewpoint of Structural Integration, tooth and jaw orthopaedics is only wise when absolutely necessary.

One should also remember that a correction of the biting

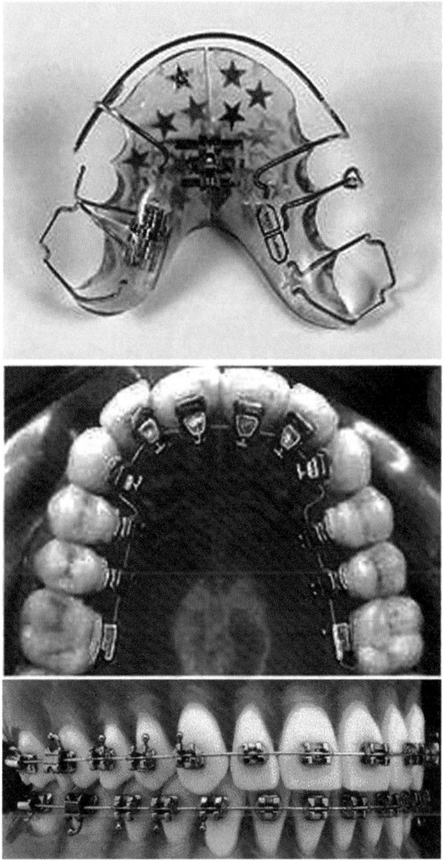

Fig. 16 Removable brace (above); fixed brace (middle and below)

position of the jaw and tooth position in the jaws usually is not a localised problem. Throughout life, the position of the teeth, facial skull and base of the skull can change. They adapt to postural load of the body and head. The bite is always also an expression of the dynamics and statics of the whole body. The state of the whole body can be responsible for deviations to the side when opening the jaw. It is more sensible to steer against malformation and correct with Structural Integration and osteopathy.

Spine

Ideally, the spine is lightly S-curved from the ninth year of age onwards. The load on the spine is in this way optimally distributed and absorbed. Frequently, this S-curve is too strongly developed or not developed enough. In the first case, the bending curve in the cervical spine and the lumbar (lordosis) area are exaggerated as well as the curves in the thoracic and sacral area (kyphosis). This group of people have a hollow back associated with a pelvis that is tilted forwards and down. In the neck and lower lumbar region the spine is *in front* of the line of gravity. This is because the chronically shortened tissue holds the tension curve. In this way, the weight of the upper body, above all the chest and the head, do not have enough support from below. These facts explain the frequently occurring tension pain in the thoracic area or in the transitional area to the lumbar region.

Altering the tension relationship in the back musculature alone is inadequate. The mentioned position of the pelvis must also be considered. The sacrum, which is tilted forwards and down with the pelvis also pulls the lumbar area with it. As long as the pelvis is not in a more horizontal postion, the back problems will not decisively improve.

If the S-curve is too weak and the spine too straight it loses its´ flexible adaptability towards load. This configuration also means that the weight of the chest and shoulder girdle has not enough support from below because the pelvis and sacrum are tilted backwards and down. Additionally, serious problems arise in the transitional area between the lumbar region and the sacrum if the 5th lumbar vertebra is forwards out of alignment. Here, slipped disc problems often arise in adulthood.

Such weak points and similar ones in the spine are subject to pronounced wear and tear as a person grows older. The oscillation permeability of the spine and the organism as a whole is decisive for the actual demands that are made on a spine.

If we consider walking under this aspect: The foot that is put on the ground brings the body weight initially down and counter pressure from the floor is elicited. This counter pressure swings like a wave throughout the organism. Precondition is of course, that this action of force is absorbed flexibly in the whole body and transmitted. (For example: the fibula bone of the lower leg is acting like a shock absorber partially absorbing and transmitting the counter pressure from the ground. This bone can only fulfil this function optimally if is „swims" freely in the surrounding tissue.)

If some joints are too flexible and others, in contrast, not flexible enough to let an undisturbed transmission occur, then the joints which are instable anyhow become overstrained. For example, if the thoracic spine is rigid and tight, the 5th lumbar vertebra and sacrum instable, then the latter will be repeatedly engaged in the rebound. A degenerative and often painful development sets in.

Overmobile segments of the spine can be relieved by making less mobile body regions more mobile again. In addition to this, the structural relationships of the pelvis and legs, which hold the whole structure, must be worked upon.

Spinal damage and damage to the feet is a topic which is hardly spoken about. Many school children suffer from back ache due to poor posture. 27% of the children aged between 6 - 12 years suffer from back ache, from 13th year upwards it is 50%.) Along with passivity (sitting too often too long), too heavy school satchels and back packs are responsible for this. Poor carrying habits also play a role.

A model project in which doctors in 2003 weighed the satchels of 312 primary school children on Budenheim in Germany gave cause for concern. On average, the satchels weighed 5-6 kilos which is much too heavy for a child which only weighs 30 – 40 kilos itself.

Let's take a look now to some special pathologies related to the spine:

Morbus Bechterew

Bechterew is a spinal disease involving an increasing curvature and stiffening of the spine starting from the lumbar region. According to *Prof. Dr. Edward Senn* who is a specialist in this area, there are three main treatment targets: 1) improving the body structure, 2) maintenance of function (mobility, respiration) and 3) learning psychophysical coping strategies. Experience shows that Structural Integration is especially suitable for achieving the first two targets if one is prepared to consider a long period of treatment. A better, more erect posture and flexibility is achievable in many cases.

Even if expectations have to remain modest, much is still gained if the ossification process can be slowed down or stopped. This target is however only realistic if Structural Integration is incorporated in a larger context including a change of diet, exercise, and where appropriate, psychotherapy.

Morbus Scheuermann

This spinal disease occurs during the prepuberty growth spurt. Wedge-shaped deformation of the front parts of the thoracic vertebrae lead to a rounded back due to the effect of gravity. Several contributing factors may be relevant here: Hormones, inheritance of damaged growth areas or if the child feels pressurized to „grow up too soon". (Fig.17).

As always when dealing with a rounded back, the key to change lies not in treating the back but in lengthening shortened tissue structure: the front of the torso (stomach muscles), iliolumbar muscles, diaphragm and the ligaments in the chest etc.

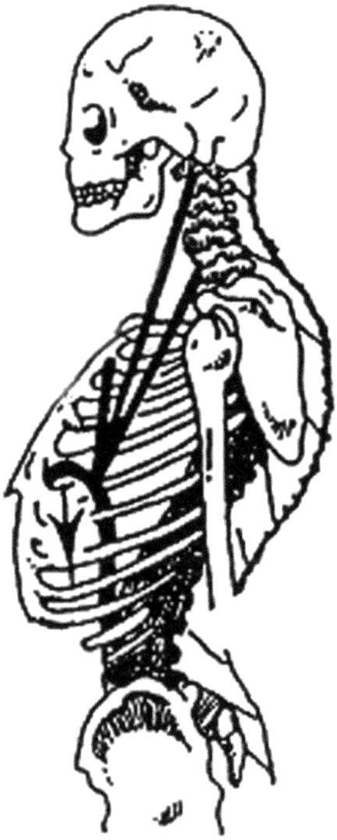

Fig. 17. Ligaments in the chest which suspend the diaphragm (and heart)

Torticollis - Wryneck

The cervical spine is fixed in a chronic flexion combined with a twist and a light over extension. At the same time, the 11th brain nerve maybe over stimulated.

There is no clearly defined cause for this in many ways puzzling set of problems. One however finds one or more of the following factors that may occur combined and hence influence one other:

- Outcome of a severe shock
- Outcome of serious dental treatment
- Eye problems can play a role
- Tense tissue in the head area
- Over tension in the supporting ligaments on one side of the lungs
- Perhaps an anatomical spinal deformation or calcification of a spinal disc
- The outcome of tuberculosis or arthritis
- Spastic as a result of a prenatal brain damage

Traditional medicine offers a rather short-sighted approach: The transection of the Sternocleido-mastoideus muscle on one side between the cranium and collar bone. This procedure is however, pointless because basic problems are not considered in the treatment and the symptoms hence soon reoccur.

Structural Integration (SI) can be helpful for many of the above listed potential causes: Applicable areas for SI are primarily: promoting the subtle mobility of cranial bones, improving the quality of the myofascial tissue between the cranium and the cervical spine, the same with the fascia in the neck and specific muscles on the side of the neck and the supporting ligaments for the lungs in the neck area. In addition, general relaxation of the vegetative nervous system helps and SI also cultivate self perception via training movement and posture. If the cause appears to be severe trauma, a combination of SI and trauma therapy is advisable.

Scoliosis

Someone with a scoliosis has a spine curved to the side (sidetilt) and rotated in the opposite direction. (Fig. 18). Only in the neck area do the twist and curve go in the same direction. The thoracic spine is usually flattened – the opposite of a rounded back. The rotation in the thoracic spine is stronger than in the lumbar spinal which crates a protrusion in the rib area.

Being born induces a mild scoliosis in everyone. If it remains marginal it does not become a problem and remains inconspicuous. Only when aggravating influences manifest is the boundary to abnormality stepped over. As so often, the transition is blurred.

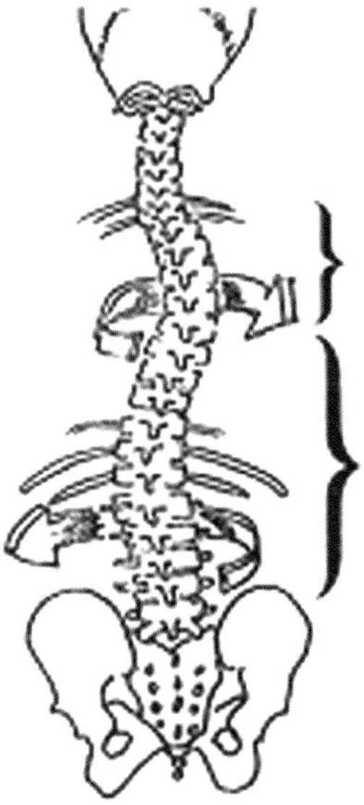

Fig. 18 Biomechanics of Scoliosis

An early scoliosis begins at the age of 5-7 years and boys suffer more frequently than girls. A preadolescent or adolescent scoliosis develops at the age of 10 – 12 and 95% of the affected are girls.

We distinguish two types of scoliosis:

a) *Idiopathic* Scoliosis includes aprominent hip but the sides of the pelvis are level.
If a double S-curve exists, the protrusion in the rib area is often absent.

Causes:

- Problems with the spine can start in the womb. It may also start during birth due to deformation of the cranium which is then „relayed" down the spine.
- KISS-Syndrome: Oblique presentation (See there)
- The child has to grow up too fast. This results in the bones growing more quickly than the muscles and the spine bends as a result.

- ➢ Problems with the organs. For example, during the embryo phase the stomach does not move from the middle to lateral and causes as a consequence a bending of the thoracic spine to the left.
- ➢ Metabolic disorders (rickets)
- ➢ Accident or an operation
- ➢ Inflammation of the thorax during childhood
- ➢ Cross-eyes can also be causative

b) *Static scoliosis*, hardly any rotation or protrusion in the rib area.

Causes:

- ➢ Asymmetrical pelvis position due to apparent or seeming difference of leg length
- ➢ Hip dysplasia (see there)
- ➢ Deformation of the thorax

The two standard therapies of traditional medicine are the corset or operating along with physiotherapy. Experience proves a corset to be contra productive because it makes the whole torso immobile and limits the proprioception of the people wearing one. An operation is not without risk and frequently the scoliosis just reappears on the other side a few years later.

Structural Integration works on an existing scoliosis with following aims:

- Improving the balance between both sides of the body.
- Facilitating movement and permeability of the whole organism.
- Normalising the lordosis and kyphosos curves by lengthening the shortened tissue structures. This lengthening can reduce the rotation of the vertebrae and so flatten the side curvature. A scoliosis with an especially long curve has a good prognosis. (Fig.19).

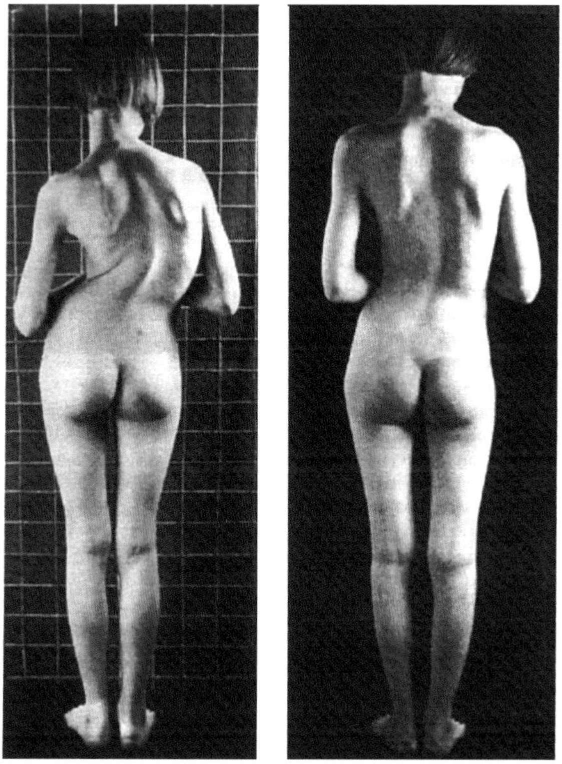

Fig. 19 A girl with scoliosis before and after a combined treatment with SI and osteopathy within 2,5 years

Important aspects of treatment are:

- Creation of an optimal balance between ventral and dorsal sides of the body; decompression of the spine and back and the sides of the torso and thorax.
- Better support of the torso via the legs (and arms).
- Optimizing the subtle cranial bone movement.
- Where necessary, releasing of connective tissue structures in the abdomen and thorax.
- Freeing the neck and achieving an optimal mobility between the head and first cervical vertebra.

One must treat a scoliosis until growth has ended. One should point out to a young person who feels him/herself to be ugly or worthless because of a scoliosis that one cannot see the spine from without but only movement. Perhaps the sufferer feels under pressure to hold him/herself straight. This leads to unnecessary tension. If is helpful to remember that the spine is not identical with the inner vertical axis.

Following recommendations are helpful if you have a child with a scoliosis:

- If the child has a static scoliosis due to one leg being shorter than the other get the child to wear a waist-high soft wollen sock on the shorter leg. This stimulates leg growth.
- All exercises which correct the subjective perception of „straight" are helpful. (Balancing something on the head, sitting on a ball with hanging legs, skiing, etc.)
- Swimming in crawl and certain other exercises from *Eurythmy*

Hip Dysplasia

This disorder involves a (usually one-sided) insufficiently developed hip bone socket. The latter being often too small and the femoral head (which may also not have the right form) cannot maintain a stable hold in the hip socket. The hip dysplasia is often coupled with a mis-alignment of the femoral head. Baby girls, who were born in a breech position, are most frequently affected.

Diagnostic signs for a developmental dysplasia of the hip are:

- One sided resistance to abduction
- The gluteal fold differs on each side of the buttocks
- Asymmetry in the contours of the pelvis, different lengths of the thighs

School medicine usually offers following treatment: Traction, a harness, braces or splint, plaster cast, operative correction of the neck of the femur and correction of the hip bone socket. Apart from the fact that these measures are unpleasant for the child, they also have many disadvantages with relation to the structural and movement development of the child. Bow legs can result; the knees and feet can develop faulty positions and spinal problems can also ensue.

Before any of the above measures are considered, one should view the possibilities of Structural Integration. These children frequently have shortened adductors and blocked iliosacral joints (the joint between the sacrum and ilium).

Legs and feet

Following a Structural Integration session, 10 year old Florian said to his mother: „I´m walking more lightly. From the inside, I can´t say how exactly."

Let us look more closely at some of the problems in this area:

The Legg-Calvé-Perthes Disease

This disease occurs in boys between the ages of 6 – 14 years and involves a painful degeneration of the upper end of the tibia. This hinders the growth of the tibia. The disease can become chronic and affect other bones. Example femoral head: Alteration of the bone socket and compression of the hip joint and that half of the pelvis. School medicine offers an operation as treatment or traction of the bone lasting a year.

In some cases, Structural Integration can bring the degeneration to a halt and reinitiate bone growth. What is important is the decompression of affected joints and segments and in the surrounding areas.

The boy Tim Barrett (who can be seen in Fig. 1 on p. 9) had this disease at the age of seven and was treated in the sixties of the last century by Ida Rolf. At the age of nine he could surf and won competitions at school. Today he works as a carpenter and has two children.

Foot Deformations

Usually, **flat feet** with a thickened ankle are not normally developed feet which have then sunken but rather underdeveloped children´s feet that have never developed an arch. Flat feet belong to the developmental phase in which a child cannot yet walk and is normal. Some feet seem to remain in this developmental phase. Structural Integration can initiate the development even if the results can be more felt than seen. The development of visibly higher arches takes time.

Insoles are not really helpful for a structural renewal because the difficulties lie not locally in the foot but rather in the unbalanced tension patterns in the myofascia of the lower leg. Additionally, insoles hinder the relearning of walking patterns on the neural and proprioceptive level.

A **club foot** involves the foot structurally being in a supination and adduction position (the foot is turned up and out and positioned inwards.) This difficulty is not easily resolved with Structural Integration. However, it can be helpful to release the often present blocked joints - the iliosacral joints and the joint between the occiput and first vertebra. The back and the hardened and shortened front side of the foot should also be dealt with.

Pigeon feet can develop structurally or from a bony malformation. This can be tested by seeing if the foot can be brought into a normal position. If this is possible, then treatment will be successful. In addition, the outer arch of the foot should be repeatedly stroked lightly. This stimulates reflexes which improve the tonus. If the cause is bony growth deformation, one should observe how the child deals with the situation. An operation may be unavoidable.

One should note that walking barefoot is advantageous for the development of healthy feet.

Knee disorders

Problems in this area are often connected to the fact that the hip, knee and foot joints are poorly aligned. It may be that the knees are continually being overstretched or in an X position. This causes continual uneven strain on the joint and partial wear.

Differing leg length

It is often not easy to determine whether one leg really is *anatomically* shorter than the other. This is because there is often no true difference in the femur or tibia length but the hip joint is compressed or one foot has sunken arches. Both can lead to a leg becoming *functionally* shortened.

The disadvantages of insoles that have been mentioned in connection with flat feet are also valid regarding functionally shortened legs. The real difficulty is often not taken into account. Instead of solving a problem, new problems are created. In only the rarest cases are insoles unavoidable.

Structural Integration can help people with legs of different length whether the cause is functional of anatomic. The associated problems such as back ache, a blocked sacrum or spinal changes can be avoided. Stance and gait become more balanced. Quite often, affected children become emotionally more relaxed, less fixed on their targets because the do not have to psychologically compensate so much within themselves.

Wearing a soft woollen leg on the thigh in the night on the shorter leg stimulates growth.

The child walks on tiptoes

In certain circumstances the child will grow out of it by the age of 6. If not, various causes should be considered. It may be a relieving posture following an accident. Perhaps the child is a sugar-junkie. A tactile hypo- or hypersensitivity may also be the cause (see page 79).

In any case, it is important that the shortened myofascia that have developed in the leg are dealt with.

Different ways of walking can be shown to the child („you can walk like this, or like that ..."). Images are helpful here such as a canary, a giraffe or a ballet dancer who walks following the performance using her whole foot to the public to take a bow.

Oblique presentation in babies (KISS-Syndrome)

A baby presents with following typical symptoms:

- asymmetric cranium and facial scoliosis
- scoliosis in the torso and a wry neck
- asymmetric pelvis
- blocked joint between the cranium and atlas (first vertebra) and between sacrum and pelvis. These factors often develop prior to birth and are frequently accompanied by a dysfunction of the spine and the uppermost ribs
- signs similar to hip-dysplasia: one sided resistance to abduction
- The gluteal fold differs on each side of the buttocks
- asymmetry in the contours of the pelvis, different lengths of the thighs
- abnormal kinesiological reactions

Along with Osteopathy, Structural Integration is a method which can be very helpful to resolve the problems.

Aftermath of accidents and operations

Three examples of structural accidents and accidents to do with mobility:

Peter (age 19) had a motorbike accident. He fell under the machine with his left hip. This caused his pelvis to become pushed to the right and the left side of his torso to shorten.

Marisa (age 7) went over her foot with a heavily loaded wheelbarrow. She suffered a foot deformation as a result and could neither walk on her toes as a result nor roll off her foot normally whilst walking.

Structural Integration helped both to overcome the problems due to their accidents.

Florian fell at the age of 14 onto a piece of glass. The wound was deep and had to be sown. Following the accident, he often had pain in his calves, knees and back. In addition, he continually walked on his toes. Through Structural Integration he learnt to use his whole foot when walking. He developed a more self-confident demeanor (!). The pain vanished.

Florian´s case is typical: Following an accident relieving postures develop that remain even when the injuries have healed. These postures have the tendency to distribute weight unevenly with unbalanced patterns of movement and also tend to become ingrained the longer they exist. It would be helpful if rehabilitation programmes would consider structural treatment to compensate such developments.

The same applies to operations. For example, a kidney which is removed from one side has an effect on the whole of the abdomen. The removal of the appendix also influences the tissues which lie more deeply which also influences the lumbar region.

3. Diseases and Symptoms

In the following chapter I will consider the contribution that Structural Integration can make towards alleviating diseases that does not (or only partially) have to do with the locomotor system.

Asthma

An over reaction to viruses, bacteria, poisons or allergens in the air, food, building materials or plants is the physiological background of asthma. The lung tissue becomes inflamed and damaged (which can be determined in some cases in a blood count) and scar tissue can form in the connective tissue. This causes hardening and thickening of the tissue connected with mucus production. The bronchioles become narrowed which causes muscle spasms due to nerve stimulation.

Breathing out – and hence breathing in – is difficult for people who suffer from asthma and for this reason many tend to pull up their shoulders und over use their chest muscles whilst breathing. This can cause pain in the ribs and sternum. Some asthma sufferers can often not even complete a sentence without pausing for breath. Their pulse rises due to fear of lack of air and due to lack of oxygen. Certain medications aggravate this effect.

Relevant asthma sprays aggravate the symptoms in the long term and weaken the liver and can cause osteoporosis. Cortisone is especially damaging regarding side effects if used frequently over a long period of time: The tissue is no longer viable and loses pain sensitivity. Reduced resistance to infection, stomach ache or discomfort, acne, disturbed vision, headaches, menstrual problems, nausea, tiredness, growth disorders in children, irregular pulse, weight gain can accompany it's use.

What causes asthma? The number of asthma sufferers in industrialised countries is much higher than in Asia, Africa or South America. Among the reasons are the following aspects: The natural production of Interleukin-10, an immune hormone, becomes disturbed due to infection avoidance from immunisation and use of antibiotics. A child´s immune system needs contact to various germs to develop effectively. If this contact is missed, the child becomes more susceptible to allergies. Children who have been through at least two viral infections in their first year of life suffer only half as often from asthma than children who have had only one or no infections during this phase of life.

It may be that air pollution is not solely responsible for an increase in allergy. Allergy was less prevalent in the German Democratic Republic although the air pollution was higher and following reunification of the two German states the occurrence of hay fever in the former GDR area rose.

Causative factors seem to be: a germ free environment, avoidance of all types of dirt and a comprehensive innoculation programme. (The innoculations against Tetanus, Polia and Diptheria are important and with few side-effects.). The immune system develops overreactions to several substances which can be expressed by way of skin eczema, hay fever and asthma.*

However, psychological causes should not be underestimated: suppressing feelings of frustration, animosity and anger, lack of body contact (longing for love and tenderness). Sometimes there is a lack of body contact with the mother. ** Other possible themes are dominance and fear born out of compulsive inability to release (not being able to let go and to have an emotional release.)

---

*Sources: *Spiegel* Online, *Spiegel* 19/2003, *Natur* (Special publication on immune defence 1989), *Science*, *British Medical Journal* and the *Institute for Tropical Medizine Uni-Clinics Tuebingen, Germany*.

**See *Literature*: A.Montagu, Koerperkontakt, p.158-162, p.164-169 and 218

Structural Integration influences various aspects of the illness:

- The body contact during the manual work can partially compensate deficiencies.
- Breathing out can be encouraged which improves breathing in and helps releasing mucus.
- Widening the chest and releasing the back enlarges the lung capacity.
- Specific techniques support the relaxation of the vegetative nervous system and open narrowed or blocked inner areas.
- Hand in hand vegetative normalization and working on tissue can improve the flow of energy through tissue which has been disturbed by cortisone.

Following hints regarding breathing are helpful for parents to give children who are in treatment:

- Breathe in for 7 heartbeats and breathe out during 9 heartbeats (feel the pulse).
- Asthma sufferers breathe high into the chest and hardly use their diaphragm. Practise breathing into the abdomen for example by lying weights or the hands on the abdomen.
- Become aware that one can only breathe as much in that one has previously breathed out.
- The child should practise breathing out with lips pressed together which supports long and even expiration.
- If the child suffers from panic attacks encourage the child to „breathe into the feelings". Alternatively, he may sit with the back facing a wall and with his hands wrapped around his knees to increase a sense of safety and security and breathe in against the wall and floor.
- Avoid the cold and do not participate in stop and go sports.

Face blindness

People who are face blind cannot recognize faces. They can only identify people via recognition of a voice. Sufferers going by do not look others in the eyes and are therefore judged to be arrogant and moody or wrongly diagnosed as autistic.

About 2% of the German population are afflicted. In half the cases the disease is inherited to the offspring.

During Structural Integration the children can be encouraged to increase their ability to recognize people via their gesticulation, body language and body structure.

Headaches

Body structure factors are also frequently relevant here.

For example, if the joint between the cranium and first cervical vertebra is compacted due to shortened muscular and connective tissue, the carotid artery can become compressed. If this is the case, this vessel puts pressure on the suboccipital nerve which increases the congestion.

If the curvature of the neck is too prominent this can also lead to headaches due to disturbance of the circulation in the spinal artery. Displacement of these vertebrae limits free blood circulation and can cause headache.

Headaches are often the aftermath of accidents, for example a whip lash injury. Following the healing of ligaments, blood vessels and muscles structural displacement of the head, neck, shoulders and spine often remain.

Further causes of headache are:

- poor posture
- hardening of the mastication musculature
- mal positioning of the jaws
- limitation of the subtle cranium bones

- If the Ligamentum nuchae (the tendon in the neck) is shortened then the head of the child is pulled backwards. This occurs when the bones grow faster than the connective tissue. The occipital joint becomes compressed.
- sinus problems
- neuralgia
- metabolic disorders
- chemical toxication from the environment and/or nutrition
- food allergies
- not drinking enough
- inflammation of specific areas of tissue
- school stress
- pressure from parents
- family or parental conflict
- noise
- lack of movement due to much traffic, highly built up areas
- lack of sleep
- too many sweets
- excessive TV and computer consumption
- long periods of use of analgesics
- possible but rare: brain tumour

Tension headaches are felt on both sides of the head but migraines only on one side and are often accompanied by nausea. During a migraine attack neurological disturbances can manifest (perception may be disturbed, numbness in the limbs). Tension headache and migraine may occur at the same time.

The cause of migraine is typically:

- an inherited tendency plus learning by imitation from the parents

- suppressed emotions and aggression, family and school conflict, lack of ability to assert oneself, lack of time for oneself
- trauma (immediately or up to 1 – 1,5 years prior to developing migraine.) The child often freezes into a combination of worry and anger.
- blocked joints in the neck, cranium and the joint between the occipital joint and atlas (first vertebra)

It is obvious that many causes of headache stem from body structural factors. For this reason Structural Integration is an essential approach to alleviate these kinds of problems. Due to the multitude of causes for headache a combination of therapies like homeopathy, Biofeedback, change of diet, analgesics with only one active substance, pain therapy should be considered.

It is interesting but not surprising to observe how the mood and behaviour alters when structural and vegetative causes of headache are conquered. Parents frequently report how their children become easier in themselves and also more talkative.

Overweight

Overweight among children and young adults is an increasing problem. The numerous causes are social, educational and psychological ones.

Treatment is for that reason complex. Obviously diet plays a central role. Structural Integration can play a key role alongside other approaches like psychotherapy, dance therapy etc.

In this context let me mention several essential characteristics of overweight young adults:

The complete dorsal side of the body is hardened because of carrying the overweight. The gait is robot-like, the legs being moved as if by the arms and feet. On the one hand, overweight children and young adults are lethargic with respect to movement on the other hand they are loaded with inner energy. The body structure is almost always the same: a hollow back, a pelvis that is tipped forwards and down, x- legs and flat feet.

Spastic brain paralysis

A spastic motor paralysis can occur prior or during birth. Normal nerve impulses are often being transmitted but appear to be limited due to shortening or hardening of connective tissue. In less complicated cases Structural Integration can alleviate sysmtoms. Deep lying myofascial tissue structures which are often very hardened are then stretched and the stretching reflexes of the antagonistic muscles can be reactivated with gentle brushing techniques.

Tactile Hypo- and Hypersensitivity

A need to be touched and held is being expressed in hyposensitivity. Children suffering from this repeatedly run into people or objects.

Hypersensitive children avoid touch, have an aversion to socks and shoes and prefer loose clothes. They have an aversion to garments with too long arms or trouser-legs. Neither do they enjoy playing with plastercine or painting with finger paints.

A child can suffer from both states at the same time. In both cases brushing the skin and a myofascia treatment is helpful.

Visual and hearing system disturbances

Problems with the ears and eyes can be a consequence of displaced cranial bones or cervical vertebrae resulting from disturbed nerve transmission and restricted circulation.

Weak sight can result from holding the head to one side whereby the visual system is used in an unbalanced manner and loses acuity. Another reason for vision difficulties can be a slight displacement of the sphenoid bone of the head.

Crossed eyes (strabismus) are usually the result of birth complications and are frequently accompanied by various bodily deformations.

- To achieve a middle field view the child tries to bring the fixing eye to the central axis of the body via a head positioned to the side and tilted. This may lead to a scoliosis.
- Lack of flexibiliy of the joint between the occipital bone of the head and the first vertebra.
- Shortening of the cervical and thoracic spine (extended head position).

These stuctural disturbances can lead to poor circulation (compressed arteries), loss of free breathing, sinking of the sternum, headaches, problems with concentrating and general nervousness.

Many children and young adults suffer from damaged hearing that needs treatment and the tendency is rising. The main cause is noise in the child´s leisure time: loud computer games, loud music, loud toys, etc. (*Medicine-Worldwide* 2004)

Chronic ear infections can lead to a disturbed flow of lymph and hence congestion in the pelvic area, chest, neck and the upper shoulder area.

Craniosacral techniques are generally helpful when combating earache.

4. Psychological Processes

Tension, lack of stability or flexibility as well as neurovegetative functional disturbances are often accompanied by inner cramps, depression, loss of feeling, fear, sleeplessness, hyperactivity and other phenomena. Structural Integration (SI) and the somatic approach can stimulate healing self-regulating processes.

Certain repetitive emotional states manifest themselves in posture and language. The converse is also true: Malposture, if repeatedly taken on, coagulate to structure and moulds the emotional experiencing world of a person. SI can initiate a retuning process.

SI cannot replace psychotherapy. Nevertheless, many children and young adults experience a healing process which corresponds with a psychotherapeutic treatment, for example:

- Deadlocked psycho-physical patterns of behaviour loosen up and open up new possibilities of dealing with the challenges of life.
- SI increases the stability of the legs and feet and hence leads literally to the person becoming more „down to earth". This creates more trust in the ability to stand on one's own feet. A more down to earth and realistic perception of one's surroundings also develops.
- A more sensitive perception of one's own limitations and a more mindful dealing with one's own body can be established.
- Frequently, a more intensive inner life along with the contact to one's needs is strengthened.
- Metabolism improves as the „permeabiltiy" of the connective tissue and it's basic substance benefits the physiological fundamentals of a balanced psyche and a healthy immune system.

Similarly to processes on the somatic level which had become stuck and can be revived, Structural Integration (SI) appears to stimulate developments on the psychological-cognitive level. Downright maturation processes can be provoked through SI.

Physical handicaps such as a sunken posture, a clumsy gait or an awkward manner can, especially for children, create uncertainty and feelings of inferiority. It is obvious what a positive physical development and change can mean for these young adults.

Scientists discovered that SI supports the right side of the brain for activities which are best managed by this

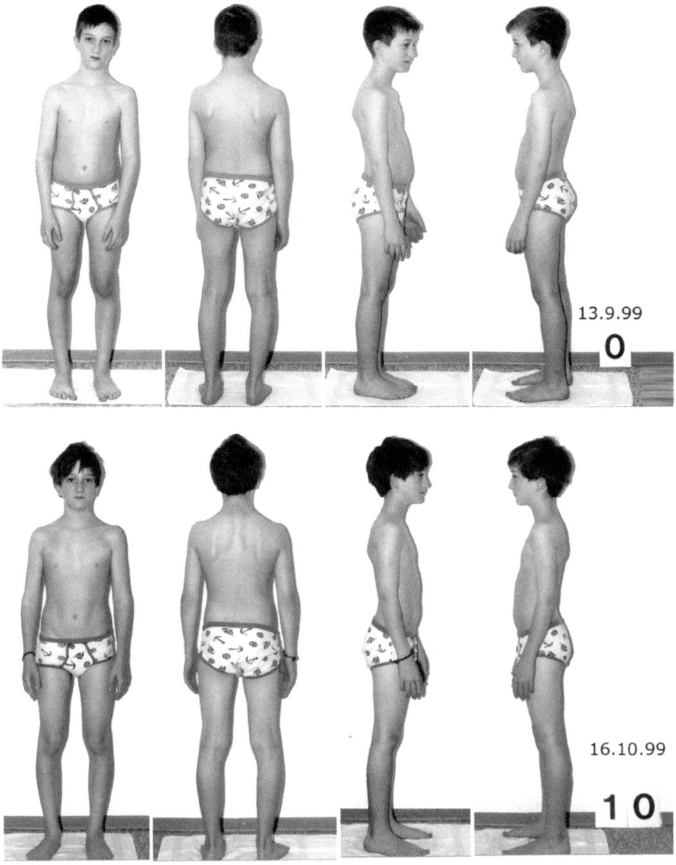

Fig. 20 Peter before and after ten sessions

side of the brain. *(Valerie Hunt et.al., A Study Of Structural Integration From Neuromuscular, Energy Field, And Emotional Approaches, Los Angeles 1977)* As is widely known, the right side of the brain processes above all intuitive, analogue, kinaesthetic thought processes and holistic thinking. In contrast, in the left side of the brain processes mainly analytical, logical thinking as well as calculating.

The same study speaks of differences in the areas of self-acceptance, presence, relationship ability and openness towards one's own feelings as compared to people who had not experienced Structural Integration.

Even if a child or young adult primarily comes because of somatic problems, a good therapist is always concurrently sensitive for psychological processes. Parents should also have this openness.

The reverse being true: if help is being sought primarily for psychological difficulties then one should clarify during the first consultation whether Structural Integration (SI) is the appropriate method or whether psychotherapy is perhaps more suitable or even if a combination of both is wise. Generally one may say: If a child senses psychological problems in the form of strong tension on the somatic level then SI with or without concurrent psychotherapy it is a good possibility for creating progress.

Conversely, it may be that a young adult may successfully go through a psychological crisis but that his body structure may lag behind. SI can here offer a rounding up or a balancing-out on the level of personal development.

In the following I would like to examine some aspects within this field more closely.

Autonomy and relationship

Alongside the centre of gravity which (except in infants) is on the level of the 3rd lumbar vertebra there exists around the 4th thoracic vertebra a second upper centre of gravity for the head, neck, chest, shoulder girdle and arms. This centre is at the same time the motor centre for the arms and hands. During movement, the centres of gravity mutually support one another. For example, when a child jumps the arms move first in the intended direction before the legs then push off the ground.

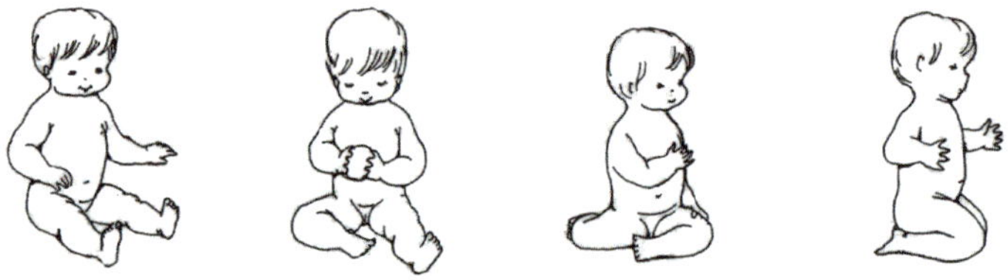

Fig. 21

One should also remember that a child first experiences the vertical from sitting and not from standing. (Fig.21).

The basic gestures of the arms are one of pushing away and gathering something in. They have a biographical significance and develop or become individually structured through the contact to the parents or figures of attachment. (Fig.22). The psychological intentions of these gestures are: receiving support through reaching out (holding and being held) and gaining autonomy through pushing away (segregation).

The boundaries to other people can, as a result of disturbed development, become too strong or too weak. In the case of weak boundaries, the person is incapable of setting limitations and adhering to them. This applies to his expression as well as through the impressions he receives from other people. Conversely, the person with over developed boundaries is incapable of taking up contact or letting him or herself be „touched" from without.

A further dimension of disturbed development may be that a child has completely given up hope of receiving support and bodily contact from his attachment figure – he has resigned.

This complex of relationship problems can be resolved during Structural Integration through manual and movement work on the connection between the chest or the heart for example. The contact to the ground as an expression of the ability to stand on one's own feet plays a role if wishing to strengthen a child or young adult.

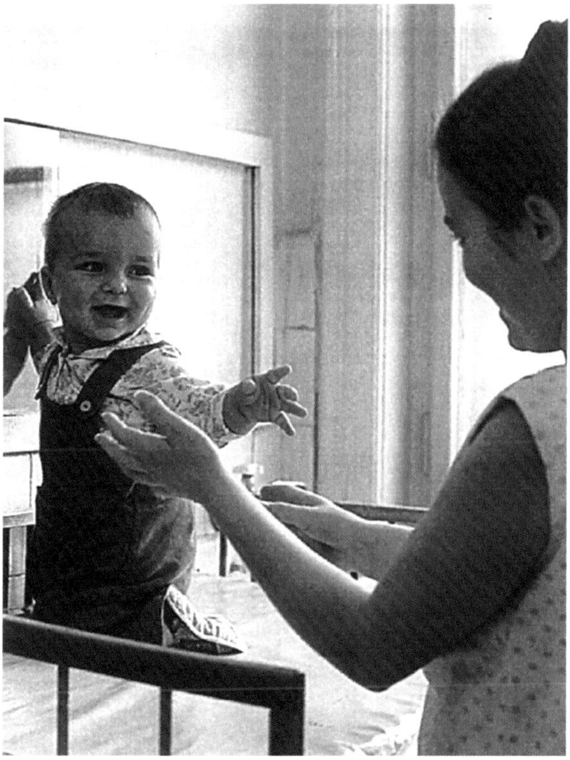

Fig. 22

Family conflicts

Loosing a parent through divorce or death is, along side with other traumata, a common cause of suffering in childhood. It manifests in a weaker form when a parent – often the father – does not have enough time for the child.

Florian, aged 6, grew up without a father. He did not show feelings of grief and sadness. This changed during the process of Structural Integration (SI). His sadness because of the missing father was clearly expressed. It was important to take the next step which was child psychotherapy.

Pascal, aged 12, had to manage a double loss. He lost his father because of the divorce of his parents and then his stepfather, who died. His mood was usually down and this manifested itself in his posture. He became aggressive following several sessions in SI, fought with his mother and showed open jealousy towards his little brother. Having gone through this phase, he generally became a happier young boy.

Miriam, aged 13, also suffered because of the divorce of her parents. This was expressed in delayed development and a migraine that she had suffered from for several years. In addition, she had poor concentration. She went through a general development during SI and her symptoms vanished. Today, 7 years later, she is still symptom free and a confident young person.

When David was 7 his father had little time for him. David was the middle child with an older and younger sister. This was difficult for him and he was aggressive and had little self-confidence. He said things like „I´m the most stupid..." He showed no sadness but was still wetting the bed at night. Various activities exhausted him. Six moths after the last SI session his mother reported that he was more lively and self-confident. He could express needs with clarity and was less aggressive. He no longer hid his sadness but showed it.

Sabine, aged 18, had a dramatic adolescence. She was training to be a nurse and had experienced the death of her father when she was 13. Depression alternated with sadness and anger. She was withdrawn and suffered from other psycho-somatic disturbances like a head tremble, bronchitis, stomach and backache. Her hearing deteriorated. She had an abortion at the age of 17. Her symptoms lessoned during SI and disappeared totally and a year later, they have not returned.

Obviously, there are times during which even in „intact" families conflicts arise between children and parents. SI can help support young persons who are maturing to mobilise their resources and enable them to emerge strengthened from such phases.

Trauma

Posttraumatic stress symptoms can result from the loss of loved ones, other physical or emotional trauma such as accidents, operations, violence, and sexual abuse. Some therapists have done specialist further trainings to be in a position to deal with such cases.

One such method is *Somatic Experiencing® (SE)*, which was developed for more than thirty years by Dr. Peter Levine out of practical studies. (Fig.23)

The stress patterns which resulted from traumatic experiences are gone into during *Somatic Experiencing* The person concerned learns to develop resources and activate the energy for self-healing to transform the experiences of previous, deep injuries.

This method is not about living out traumatic feelings but rather a step by step „new-deal" with the symptoms and bound-up energy to set it free and utilise it for a gradual self-healing process.

Fortunately, sensitivity for posttraumatic disorders in our society – especially among children – has increased. However, subtle signs are still often not noticed and therefore the appropriate treatment is not undertaken.

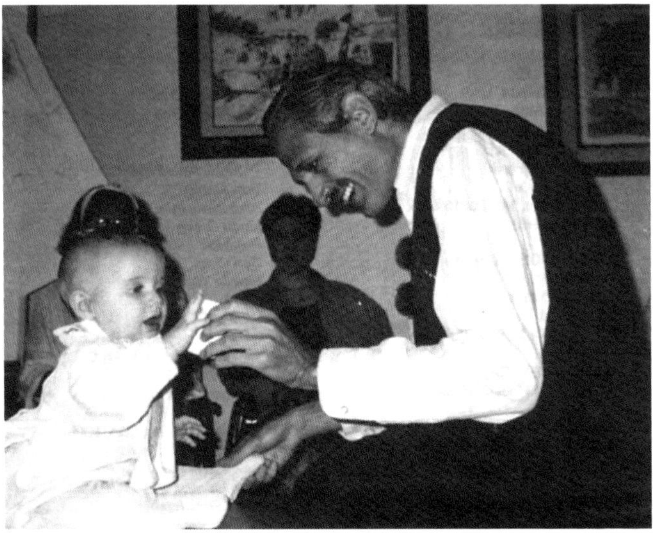

Fig. 23 Dr. Peter Levine
He was trained by Dr. Ida Rolf in Rolfing-SI. As a Biologist and Psychologist, he became a stress consultant for the NASA, the Hopi Guidance Center in Arizona and psychiatric clinics in Denmark. He works world-wide on projects to reduce chronic stress.

Varied experiences can be traumatizing:

- Intrauterine poisoning during pregnancy
- Ceaserian birth (too rapid decompression and the first long stimulation of the body is not experienced)
- lack of oxygen (birth, near drowing accidents)
- ether anaesthetization
- being attacked by animals or criminals
- sexual abuse
- natural catastrophes (earthquakes, fire, etc.)
- falling, especially from hights
- injuries and operations

- illnesses (especially with a very high temperature)
- hospitalization (immobilisation, separation, death etc.)
- loss of a loved person
- medical treatment (being strapped down, anesthetization when frightened etc.)

Signs of trauma in a child can be:

- adamant and rigid wish to control things
- regression
- uncontrolled attack of anger
- hyperactivity
- being easily scared
- reoccuring nightmares or awakening regularly, lashing out in sleep
- bed wetting
- forgetfullness, lack of concentration
- quarrelsomeness or withdrawal
- fearfullness
- being over-affectionate
- physical problems without obvious reasons

It is known that two people who experience the same traumatic situation react in different ways. Some become more traumatised than others. This depends upon how stable someone was prior to the trauma. Apart from this, it is relevant how someone manages to keep the inner and outer orientation and remain capable of being able to act. Obviously, both aspects are interrelated.

To try to find out whether unusual behaviour of a child is connected with a traumatic reaction, one can mention the relevant episode and observe the behaviour of the child. If the child reacts with strong aversion or overexcitement or a fearful flow of talking, it is a sign that a trauma could be present.

When working with children one adapts and becomes sensitive to signs which could point to a possible traumatisation. This applies to the quality of touch as well as the manual techniques which are used and the relationship quality. In the treatment process special emphasis is laid upon the child's ability to integrate change.

Generally, one can say that the greatest trauma that a person can experience is a massive breach of his or her boundaries. The result being that a traumatised child can no longer (or only poorly) sense his or her personal boundaries. In addition, the involved person often only had as an escape from the situation a partial exit out of ones own body.

Therefore every therapeutic and padagogical approach includes reestablishing sensing for one´s own boundaries. This can be accomplished by creating a safe container with the hands or with the aid of the ground or a wall or a blanket. It's also possible to achieve this goal via stimulation of processes of perception related to physical feelings, breathing, spontaneous movements, inner images, feelings and thoughts. Within the relationship between the therapist and child personal boundaries should be respected with sensitivity and the autonomy of the personal „I" strengthened.

It may be that a child has had a negative experience in the phase before it could speak. Resolving the traumatic situation can be done through subtle work on the vegetative nervous system (stress reduction) which can sometime be caught up on in a playful way.

Children can often be traumatised by situations which appear harmless to adults. In addition, children are able to successfully hide signs of traumatic reactions and prove how „tough" they are. (The latter is unfortunately frequently encouraged by adults). That is why it is important to recognize the existence of a current trauma. A glazed look, paleness, rapid, flat breathing, trembling, disorientation, and a lack of presence are typical symptoms.

Here are a few first aid recommendations following an accident or fall of a child:

1. Attend for an instant to your own reactions to avoid transferring your reactions to the child (children react with great sensitivity to the reactions of the adult present)
2. Calm the child down, take it into your arms if possible and offer warmth.
3. Be firm with the child that it takes enough time to rest in a quiet, safe place. If you have take the child into your arm, make sure you do not limit it's mobility.
4. Initially, do not talk about the accident.
5. Confirm and mirror all physical reactions regarding the accident.
6. When the first stun gradually recedes direct the child's attention gently to it´s sensations. „What can you feel in your body?" „Is there anything that does not hurt, that feels good?" Wait for a reaction. Then ask about pain and other unpleasant sensations. „Where can you sense the bad feeling?" „How does is feel in your abdomen (or elsewhere)?" Ask gently about the area, size, „colour", weight and other characteristics of the discomfort zone. Then guide the child gently back to the present moment. „And how does the bump (or what ever) feel now?"

   Take your time for quietness between the questions and give confirmation for the good, safe, strengthening sensations. The latter are the resources with which the negative feelings can be better endured. Take enough time to let a reaction cycle come to an end. The signs of such a completed cycle are: A deep, relaxed breath, lessening of trembling or crying, stretching, smiling, taking up or letting go of intense eye contact, orientation reactions. Further cycles can follow.

Attention disorders, hyperactivity

Children with attention disorders without hyperactivity have contact problems and are retarded in their development. These children with the diagnosis of attention deficit disorder (ADD) are quiet, shy and withdrawn. The explanation monopoly on this topic resides with neurologists. Findings on ADD from social psychologists, stress researchers, environmental doctors and researchers on consciousness have not been adequately considered.

It is however true that stressed children behave exactly as ADD children do. The brain chemistry of such children shows alterations which *accompany* the symptoms but which are not the *cause* of the symptoms. Henning Köhler, an experienced therapist for children and adolescents reports that, in his experience, these children possess a high introspective intelligence and are very empathic. (*Info 3*, 2002) However, this cannot be expressed due to their shyness and they therefore often land in special schools labelled as having a low intelligence.

A major problem these days is that behavioural problems due to problematic life situations or traumatic experiences, abuse or neglect are being confused with ADD. A certain proportion of cases in this field is accounted for by the „minimal brain dysfunction in children" which is caused due to lack of oxygen during birth. One must point out that many children have been diagnosed as having ADD because they are totally frustrated by today's cramped living situation and by their school situation. Their capabilities remain unrecognized and their needs not adequately considered. Because they do not feel accepted how they are.

Another common diagnosis these days is attention-deficit hyperactivity disorder (ADHD). This behaviour disorder among young people is, according to neurologists, caused by changes in the brain due to a lack of neurotransmitters such as dopamine. In the brain of ADHD children a partial system responsible for controlling drive utilising the neurotransmitter is supposedly altered. The lack of dopamine hypothesis was postulated when one discovered that symptoms improved when substances where administered which stimulate the production of dopamine. Subsequently, one searched intensively for shifts within the dopamine system and all that was then found was taken as confirmation for the hypothesis. This however, does not confirm the source of the behaviour disorder and indications that a basic genetic defect is the cause should likewise not be over-judged. All symptoms can be otherwise explained. For example, disturbances including enhanced reactions have been well documented in medical literature for many years. The list of symptoms correlates surprisingly well with that of ADHD. The same can be said for stress, lack of concentration and other states of inner disquiet caused by allergy; the transition to instability is not clearly definable.

Dr. Gerald Hüther is a doctor and Professor for Neurobiology in the psychiatric clinic at the University of Göttingen. He had previously occupied himself with experimental medicine and brain development disorders at the Max-Planck-Institute. He states that there is much evidence for the fact that „many children exist who already as newly born are considerably more awake, brighter, more curious and easily stimulated than others." (*Info 3*, 2001) These children need, according to Dr. Hüther, an especially quiet, supportive and low stimulus environment so that they can develop their potential and abilities. Lack of protection of such children from overstimulus (eg. via television or internet) can lead to a negative development. Their brain then develops in a manner which is different to that which is commonly necessary for dealing with recurring new stimuli, this includes their dopamine system.

A certain important factor which is frequently ignored in our society should also be considered. Dr. Hüther states: „In all circumstances, we must stop wishing to be as quick as possible, better, faster and more effective than others." The present trend however is marked by commercialisation and technization with increased overstimulation from the entertainment industry, increasing social coldness and loss of contact to Nature. How can children feel at home in such a world? They are all more or less under stress. They do not know where they can play. The have no free scope to move in. Their life has been flattened and straightened up and is under control. Alongside them are stressed and frustrated parents. Their small beings are being bombarded with toxins daily.

Regarding the medicinal treatment of ADHD with the drug Ritalin, Dr. Hüther says:

„The line of arguement up to now has been: The children have a deficit in their dopamine activity and this genetically caused dopamine deficit can be corrected through treatment with Ritalin.

This mechanistic attempt of an explanation has become questionable. The dopamine system could also have become overdeveloped during the first years of life. There is some new research evidence which points to this. Ritalin would then empty the dopamine resevoir and during the following hours – when the reservoir would be filled again - this system, being overdeveloped and enhancing the drive, would be switched off temporarily.

If a child has such an overdeveloped dopamine system it would make sense to administer Ritalin. If, however, the child has been misdiagnosed the normally developed dopamine system would be obstructed in its further development by Ritalin.

If this happens one sets the scene for something that only manifests itself much later (from the fiftieth year of life or later): Parkinson´s disease which is a result of a lack of dopamine activity in the brain areas responsible for regulating movement and coordination.

If children have social difficulties due to their behaviour they must obviously be helped. This otherwise has, if the situation continues, unclear impact upon their further brain development. Ritalin can apparently be so easily and effectively applied, and this has led to a lack of research and use of other therapies. More should be done in this area in the future. If everything else has been attempted perhaps there is nothing else to do apart from accepting the dangers of an as short as possible treatment with Ritalin."

However, it is important that parents do not uncritically take everything on board which is said and recommended by authorities on this topic.

If you are a parent having to deal with this topic you should seek support from paediatricians, therapists, and teachers who do not think of a disturbed dopamine system in the brain but rather a child in need of loving, empathic attention. Perhaps you should also consider a change of school. Waldorf and Montessori schools implicitly offer several things which other schools lack:

- active parental involvement and responsibility
- attention to the individual development of the pupils
- a holistic approach meaning that not only intellectual development but also the emotional aspects are regarded
- learning without fear or pressure and hence teamwork within stable classes
- many practical subjects with practical courses for the pupils
- support with development of artistic and craft abilities

As far as stress and not feeling in inner balance play a role one should not underestimate the support that Structural Integration could offer within the mosaic of possibilities that could help a child within the field of attention disorders.

Conversion of lefthandedness

Handedness is the expression of the motoric dominance of one side of the brain which is expressed in the preferred use of the contralateral hand. Probably around 30% of the population are left-handed. True ambidexterity (someone who is able to write with both hands) indicates the presence of cerebral damage. Enforced retraining from left to right is seldom these days. However, it often occurs that a child who is actually left-handed changes to the right through imitating of adults or other children.

Whatever the case, it is not that the dominance of the side of the brain alters but the not dominant side becomes overloaded, the dominant half is not challenged enough and transmission problems develop in the fibre connections between the two halves of the brain. This „knot in the brain" can bring forth following symptoms:

- Disturbances of memory and concentration (the child tires easily)
- reading and writing problems (dyslexia and musical dyslexia)
- problems distinguishing left from right
- fine-motoric disturbances (also in hand-writing)
- problems with speech, stuttering
- feelings of inferiority, unsureness, withdrawal
- compensation via hightened effort
- defiance, showing off, clowning
- bed wetting, nail-biting
- vegetative symptoms: sweating attacks, jittery eye-lids, muscular twitches, headaches, ticks and sleeping problems
- neurosis and behavioral disturbances

Whether a conversion from left to right has taken place is often difficult to determine. If a forced conversion has occurred, the memories of it are often suppressed or belittled because the memory is too painful and associated with shame. If conversion has occurred via imitation this is also difficult to ascertain because it may have taken place inconspicuously. In addition, because the problem of handedness is not widely known, behavioural problems at school and in therapy are often ascribed to other sources.

To determine handedness, minor activities with minimal influences from upbringing such as throwing dice, pivoting something, catching the teacher's eye, picking up small objects or counting beads, hammering, combing etc. should be used.

Structural Integration can help compensate the consequences of an early conversion such as vegetative disturbances, uncertainty with spatial orientation and fine-motoric weaknesses. Retraining back to left handedness is not always the right approach as this can be emotionally challenging as well as putting high demands on the nervous system.

Dyslexia

The afore mentioned child psychologist Henning Köhler says: „My experience is that many of the so called dyslexic children are those who are only really ready to learn cultural techniques such as reading and writing from the age of ten onwards. If they are not by that age yet fully traumatised with regard to reading and writing the breakthrough happens with at least 60% of the so-called dyslexics. This takes place if it is possible to approach them from their creative manuell, social and experiencing side. One is successful if the feeling is conveyed that they are learning something for life."

The others have, according to Köhler, true deficits in their fine-motoric and coordination skills. Such children must be assisted „primarily to become sure with their hands and their bodies so that they can act in balance." (*Info 3*, 2002) It is obvious that Structural Integration can be useful in improving the coordination abilities and fine-motor skills.

Anorexia and Bulimia

The young people concerned, usually girls in adolescence or post adolescence, come mainly from the middle or upper classes. They often grew up overprotected meaning that they developed bonds which were too strong. Alternatively they felt rejected by their family and consequently developed problems with bonding.

The common development is: the teenager is anorexic, then addicted to food, then has both conditions, alternating. The latter condition expresses itself with vomiting into the toilet following eating. An extreme discrepancy exists between how the young person see herself („too fat") and reality. She feels torn between thinking and feeling and this leads to auto-aggression and depression.

Bulimia seldom clears up completely because it is an addictive illness and the drug food is not completely avoidable.

Experience shows that Structural Integration presents a series of possibilities to positively influence the way a young person sees herself and hence influence the behaviour of anorexic girls. Treating the spine and the abdomen as well as integrating individual changes in an overall context of structure, movement and perception play a major role. It is useful to complement dancing or dance therapy to this.

Autism

Autism is in many ways a puzzling phenomenon. The causes of this disposition remain unclear. For this reason I will only touch a few aspects to demonstrate how Structural Integration could be helpful.

It is conspicuous that autistic children have a weak spatial orientation. One of the first symptoms being that autistic children often cannot point at something. Hence, social isolation starts or accompanies spatial isolation.

In addition, autistic babies demonstrate abnormal patterns of movement with regard to turning, sitting up, crawling and learning to walk. Could early treatment help such children?

Manual treatment using reasonable pressure which parents can also learn, specific craniosacral techniques and supporting the ability to spatial orientation has a positive effect upon the development of children.

5. Music, Dancing and Sport

Parents frequently bring their children who are learning an instrument or taking dancing lessons to Structural Integration. During dancing, sport or playing music the body serves as an expression medium.

For example, a young ballet dancer who may feel herself to be very mobile in her legs and pelvis but is dissatisfied with her expressiveness in her shoulders and chest. Such a person may wish to do something to prevent joint problems at a later stage.

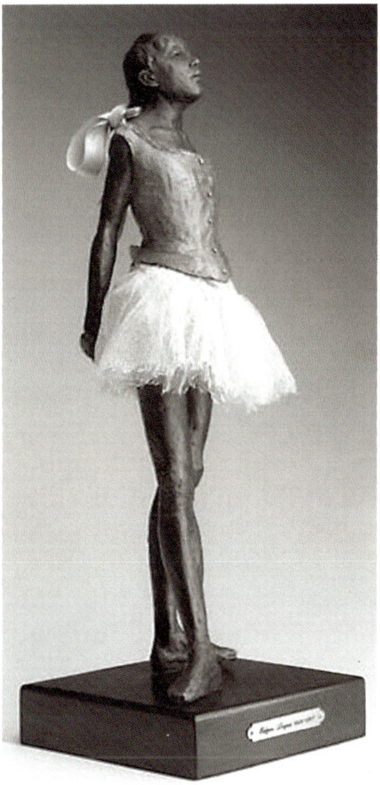

Fig. 24 The young dancer (Edgar Degas)

The physiologically problematic posture which is demanded from someone doing ballet sometimes leads to pain in the joints and a raised danger of injury. The posture includes a hollow back, legs and feet that are rotated outwards and knees that are overextended. In addition, the young person usually transfers this posture consciously or unconsciously into every day life. (Fig.24).

A young girl learns to play the violin. The position that she continuously has to adopt often leads to chronic neck and shoulder tension combined with a rotation of the trunk to the left. This not only limits well being but also artistic expression and the fine aspects of the musical tone.

A gifted young man of nineteen years plays the piano. His shoulders are tense, his wrists often pain him and he suffers from cold hands and feet. Closer inspection reveals that he sits with his back sagged backwards. Hence his shoulder girdle and arms are not well supported. The over stained shoulders are pushed forwards resulting in poor circulation of the arms and hands. When sitting like this, playing strength does not arise from the centre of the body but primarily from the arms and hands which therefore become strained. This is the cause of the pain in the wrists.

In cases such as these the aim of Structural Integration is to achieve prophylactic posture improvements and to seek for musicians and dancers possibilities to enhance expressiveness and improve litheness and permeability. This aim is obviously coupled with working on existing problems through treating the myofascial tissue.

Widespread lack of movement is common among children and young adults and has been afore mentioned in this book. It is generally accepted that sports and games are an important compensation for periods of long sitting.

Equally important however, is avoiding a too early or exaggerated achieving mindset. The not yet fully developed person cannot bear this without suffering in some way. Strongly one sided strain from sport prior to the 21st year of life causes structural and functional (joint) problems. A gymnast often has a hump around the 6th cervical vertebrae, a boxer frequently a kyphosis around the 8th vertebrae and a tennis player an overly loose spine.

This gives cause for thought. I am in no way speaking out against competitive sport but rather for putting playfulness and pleasure in the foreground.

People who do sport spend much time on developing parts of their body – stronger legs, arms, etc. What is often missing is a comprehensive perception of their body as an integrated whole utilising strength in a balanced fashion connected to greater flexibility with less use of energy but with a finer coordination.

The risk of injuring oneself during sport, e.g. during football, greatly depends upon the permeability of an individual with respect to movement impulses. Lack of mobility in the pelvis and hip joint can destabilise the knee for example. This is because lack of mobility from the hip joint has an affect on the pull and push on the knee.

Chronic problems are not infrequently the result of regular sport. In time, a bike rider will for example suffer from chronic pain in the lower back. Treating and teaching him optimal posture can help to reduce pain and at the same time increase performance. (Fig.25)

Structural Integration can improve coordination and mobility. The reason: A greater structural balance and flowing, harmonic muscle activity leads to an increase in

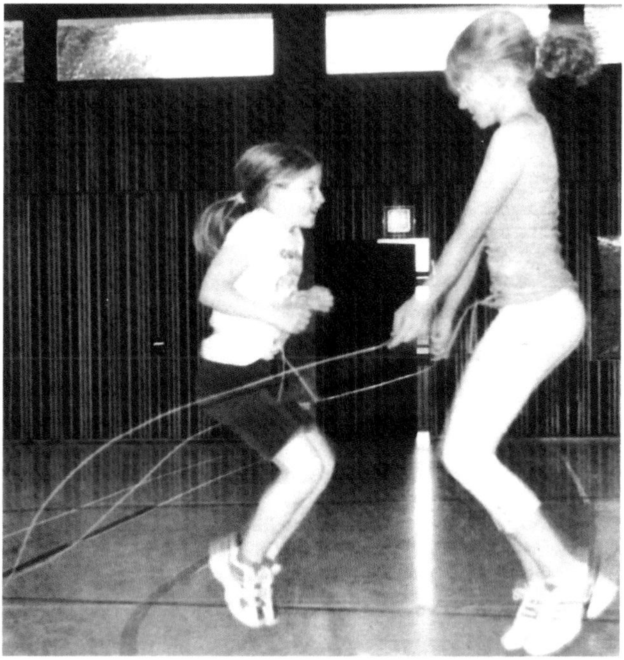

Fig. 25 Rope skipping: oeconomical (right) and unoeconomical (left) performance

lighter and more effective and graceful movement.

There are healthy and less healthy forms of sport and not each type of sport is equally appropriate for everyone.

The most optimal forms of sport are swimming and cross-country skiing because the body is used evenly in a balanced fashion. If knee problems already exist, bike riding is less demanding than other forms of sport. For children who do not have much movement and somewhat reticent emotionally, sports which have expressive movements like dancing, martial arts or ball games are extremely helpful.

If the sport demands one-sided movements such as tennis the young person should do another sport beside tennis to compensate this so that both sides of the body are used.

Certain types of sport are suitable for certain body types:

- The repetitive compressing movements of long distance runners are unsuitable for young people with compact bone structure. If the young person has little fat tissue and a good metabolism, long distance running is suitable.
- If someone has fragile bone structure contact sports could be dangerous.

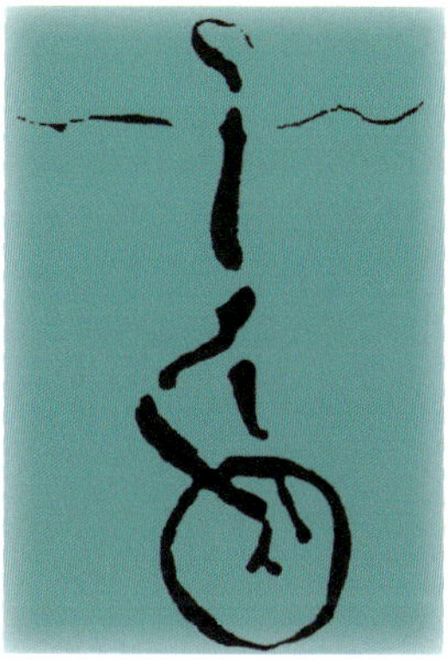

Practical Hints for Everyday Life

1. Bodily Exercises

During the process of Structural Integration the practitioner will give your child some „homework" in the form of certain bodily exercises. Irrespective of this, I explain some exercises in the following which you can now and again do with your child. In the process, please remember that playfulness goes before hard practise.

Remember to warm up prior to all stretching exercises (which should be held for at least 30 seconds) and not to hold your breath whilst doing them.

General exercises

Developing balance

- Standing on one leg
- Diagonal quadruped position (an arm and the leg of the opposite side are held horizontally)
- Balancing on an instable base (seesaw or trampoline) in sitting or standing
- Balance a bean or rice bag on the head to develop straightened alignment

Lengthening and stretching the iliolumbar musculature

Standing with the help of a stool: One leg is placed backwards (foot directed forwards, the heel lifted), the other leg with the foot directed forwards is placed on the chair. The child now moves forwards from the hips and knee which is on the stool. Avoid hollowing the back during this exercise. (Fig.26)

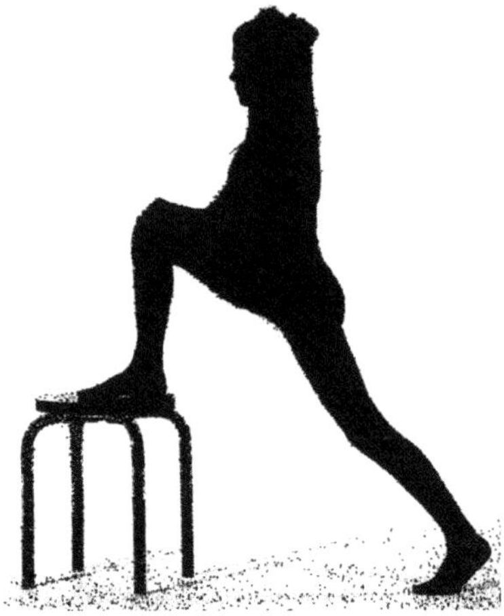

Fig. 26

Stretching the trunk and mobilising the spine

Start lying down on the side. The right leg lies stretched out and the left leg is bent and held on the floor with the hand. Slowly now turn the upper (left) shoulder with the arm to the left. The head looks towards the horizontally out stretched arm (Fig. 27). Repeat with the other side.

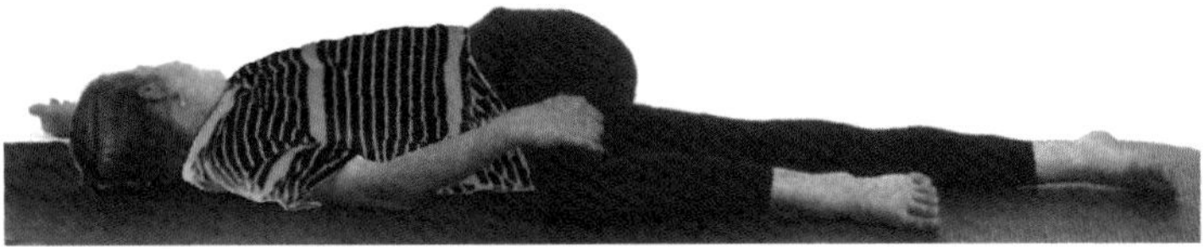

Fig. 27

Stabilising the trunk

Within orthodox physiotherapy or the fitness branch there is much talk of strong abdomen muscles or stabilising the trunk to prevent back ache. One now knows however, that in truth there is only one abdomen muscle which stabilises the trunk during great effort: The transversus abdominis. Additionally, the issue is more about activating and not strengthening this muscle which runs horizontally like a broad belt.

Pull in the navel with maximal effort towards the spine, hold this for 30 seconds and then let go. Repeat this with half the effort. If the child can do this with half the effort and keep the hollow abdomen it should breathe normally while it holds in. Start in quadruped position, and then practise with the back lent on a wall, then standing freely and then lying on the back. Do this with a leg first pulled in the direction of the chest and then stretched. Be careful not to pull the thorax up during the exercise.

Exercises for certain structural problems

A round back and collapsed thorax

➢ Place a roll or a tightly rolled up towel under the back on the level of the peak of the round back. Fold the arms behind the head and lower the shoulders slowly to the floor. Now bend a leg. Place the foot of the other leg on the knee and relax. Then repeat with the other leg. (Fig. 28)

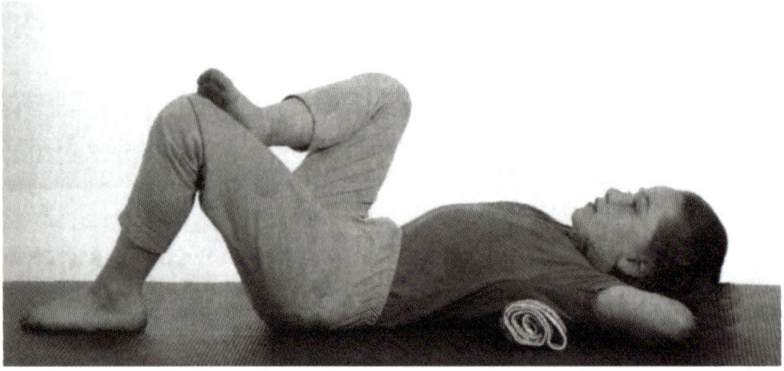

Fig. 28

➢ In a sliding position the weight of the torso lies on the lower arms. Release the abdomen and let the whole torso sag. (Fig.29)

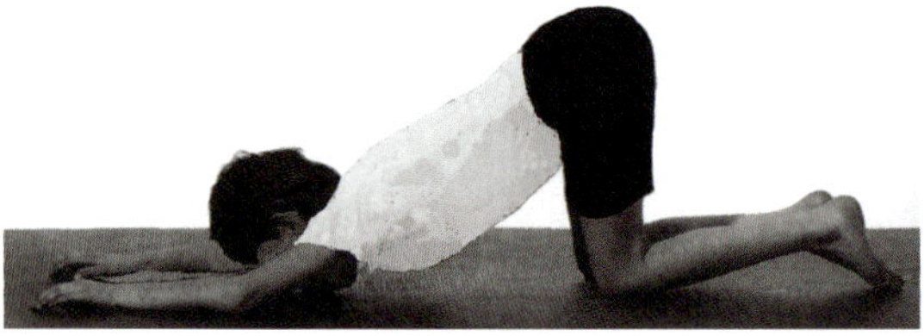

Fig. 29

Hollow back and a pelvis tilted forwards and down

➢ Lie on the edge of a table with the sitting bones in contact with the table. One leg hangs over the edge of the table, the other is bent and pulled up to the chest. (Fig.30)

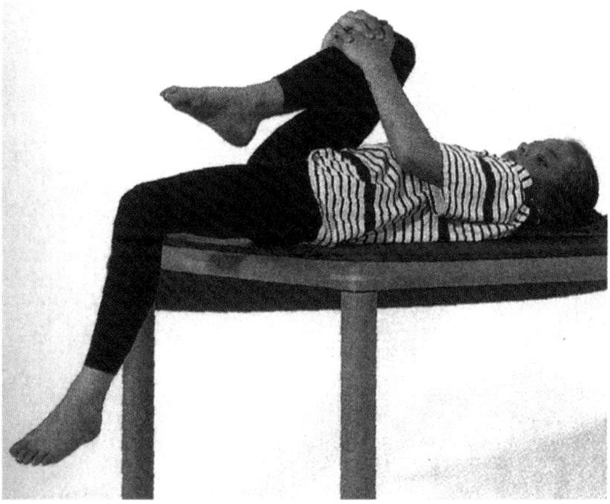

Fig. 30

➢ On the back. Pull the legs to the chest and hold them with the hands. Breathe whilst doing this into the lower back.

➢ Balance objects while standing or walking on the head. This stretches the spine.

A pelvis which is tilted back and down; over-stretched knees

The pelvis which is tilted back and down is often also pushed forwards. This structural constellation often means that the centre of the body sags forwards (see Fig.4 b, page 14). Another common pattern are overstretched knees (see Fig.4 a, page 14). For both patterns *folding bending* (Fig.31) is an especially helpful exercise.

➢ One initiates the lowering movement through yielding to ones own weight whilst bending the hip, knee and ankle joints. It is important to not pull the buttock or the sitting bones up but to let them glide backwards.

Moving upwards is initiated by letting the pelvis and sitting bones slide even further back and up a little bit while more and more weight is transferred to the legs and feet. Then one glides upwards via pushing the feet towards the floor. During the whole procedure the arms hang freely and the breastbone „looks" forwards.

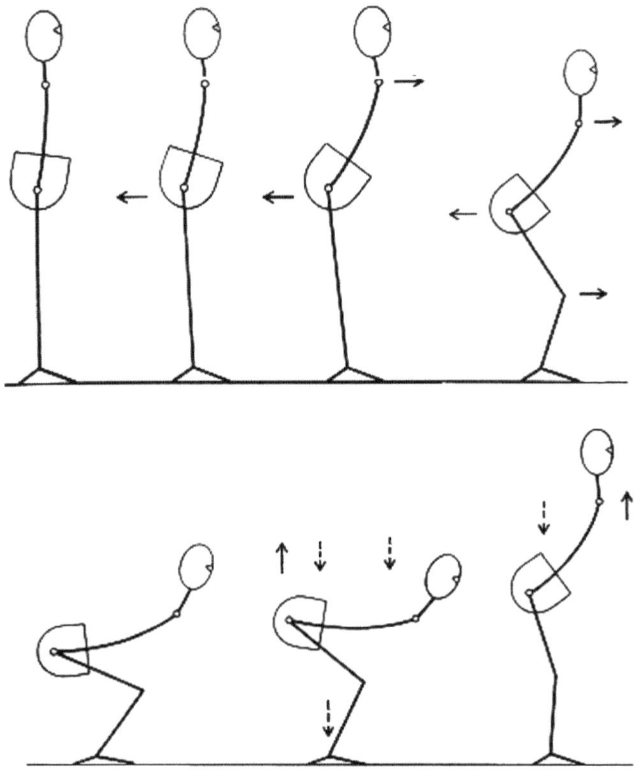

Fig. 31 Folding bending
(solid arrows: direction of movement; dotted arrows: direction of gravity)

2. Sitting , Bending and Lifting

The design of seats which take people with respect to structural aspects into consideration are still rare. This situation is especially poor in schools. Surveys show that only about 40% of children have furniture which is adequate for their age. Try out with your child prior to buying furniture which chair is best. Below you will find some helpful hints.

The height of the table should have an adequate relationship to the height of the person sitting and body size. If the table is too high then elbows or lower arms which are put on the table are pushed upwards. If it is too low, the user adopts a round back.

In general it must be said that school children do not have enough exercise or relaxation breaks. This is, however, necessary because children cannot continually concentrate and every person needs a break following a period of sitting still. Otherwise the nervous system becomes exhausted and a tendency develops to slouch in the chair.

Here are some hints for a back-friendly way of sitting that you could first try yourself and then playfully rehearse with your child. (Fig.32):

- The chair should have a height so that the knees are slightly lower than the sitting bones.
- The feet should not be too far in front or behind the knees because then support is lacking and the pelvis cannot come into the right position.
- In an optimal position the pelvis is slightly tilted forwards and down. To accomplish that one rotates the pelvis around an imaginary transverse axis which runs across the pelvis, a little bit above the hip joints. The child does this until he senses that he is sitting on the front part of the sitting bones. If you are worried that the child adopts a hollow back in this position: The fear is unfounded if the abdominal muscles are not tensed

whilst the pelvis is rolled and the back muscles remain relaxed. Some children find a wedge-shaped bolster helpful in achieving the right pelvis position.

- If the child still has a strongly rounded upper back and the lower back is too tense as a consequence: Then the child should swing the whole upper body from the hips slowly until it feels that tension in the back lessens and he is in balance.
- As the weight of the torso is now in front of the hip joints and falls down, the upper part of the body can with ease align itself upwards from the pelvis and relieve the back and make a relaxation of the neck and shoulders possible.
- Minimal movements of the back hinder a static sitting position, improve metabolism in the small muscles and the joints of the spine and encourage awareness. It is also helpful to imagine the spine as a reed or bamboo stick which gently moves in the wind.

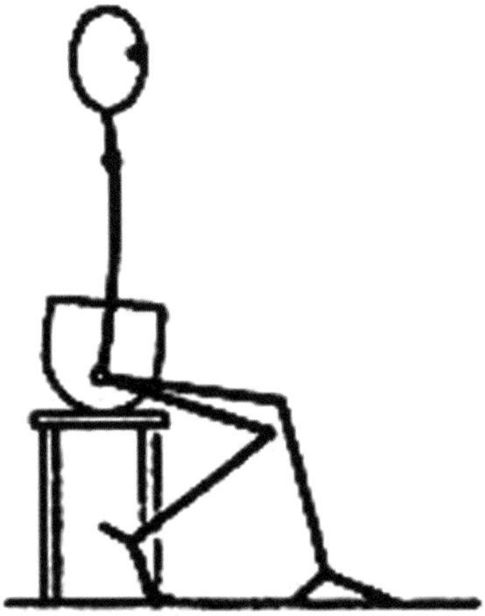

Fig. 32

- A child can move easily and ergonomically from the optimal sitting position forward or down. It is important that such a movement takes place from the hips and that the sitting bones are moved back during it. The abdomen remains relaxed so that the torso keeps a gentle forward convex curve.
- Changing sitting positions is quite normal. From time to time, a slouch is allowable. Perhaps the child can sense that a straight alignment now belongs to his „repertoire" and can be recalled at will.

Most back training schools emphasise bending knees to bend downwards and lift things. This is certainly more ergonomic than bending and lifting with a rounded back. However, the back and above all the knees can be unburdened if one performs the movement in a type of folding bending (see Fig. 33 below and Fig. 31 on p. 108)

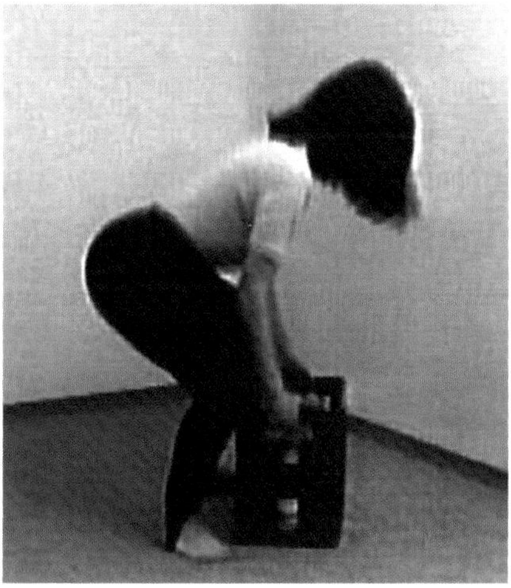

Fig. 33

The described exercise regarding bending and lifting obviously has to be modified for everyday life. Feet are usually not set parallel but one in front of each other. Sometimes the young person may feel uncomfortable with the bottom being so far back. Of course he or she should feel free to rearrange him or herself or to turn around so that the bottom is then less obvious.

3. Clothes and Shoes

Clothes should always be wide enough so that the child or young person has sufficient room to move and breathe freely and that the inner organs are not restricted in any way.

When buying shoes one can consider following points so that the feet are assisted in their work:

- Sufficient space must be available for the arch of the foot to stretch and bend.
- The shoes should allow a hinge like movement between the ankle and heel and between the middle of the foot and the toes. A few minutes walking, testing the shoes is helpful prior to deciding to buy.
- The foot bed should not press into the length of the arch of the foot which would throw the weight of the body to the outside of the foot.
- The bed of the shoes and sole should allow the foot to adapt to various surfaces and roll off easily. Wooden shoes and clogs are therefore unsuitable.
- Sandals without straps on the heel force the toes to continually hold the shoes which hinders the rolling of the feet and causes chronic shortening of the relevant muscles and tension on the calves.
- The shoes should facilitate a flowing transition from slow to fast movement. (Can the child run for the bus comfortably in the shoes?)

4. Dealing With the Television and Computer

Surveys showed that many children aged 10 have a whole line-up of equipment in their bedroom (e.g. television, computer, play station DVD player). In some areas up to 80% of boys are using the computer over 30 hours a week. These figures illustrate how important this topic is.

Computers and the television are valuable communication media and are also supportive to creativity. I wish to make clear that I do not wish to demonize them. The following information should assist you however, in appropriately judging how much and which media is good for your child.

Early and intensive occupation with modern communication technology alters the way a child thinks and perceives.

Ones relationship to time also alters. Virtual games on the screen happen very fast so that children's relationship to reality (school for example) appears to be in slow motion. This results in children continually expecting new, hyperactive and videoclip-like experiences at school.

Herta Sturm, a media psychologist, investigated how television and computer games alter mind processes a few years ago. She discovered that real life is marked by tiny breaks in activity. We take a breath in a moment of doing nothing, turn our head to adjust our view of things or move to a door or a window. In these moments we name what is occurring and integrate it in our inner world and hence prepare for what is coming. In front of a screen however, the viewer hastens from image to image, and situation to situation without time to digest. The memory takes up only diffuse emotional impressions, no self-reflection occurs and content can only be poorly recalled or not at all.

Within the context of this book, it is also interesting to note that body-related experiences cannot be made. Perception is stored in the mind but not in the body. Special courses for engineering students in the United States have already been started to compensate for lack of tactile, spatial and mechanical experiences. Prof. Henry Petroski calls these courses coaching in playing with real objects.

Many parents fear that their children will miss out in the future if they do not already learn at infants or primary school how to deal with computers. Martin Large, the English educationalist researcher rightly comments however, „a child has not missed anything if it only types it's first www at the age of 10."

It even appears that too early and excessive use of computer and television, even under the point of view of education, can be harmful. Experts complained at the annual meeting of the American *Space Foundation* 2002 that the emerging generation is not adapted to the high technology branch. Their ability to think abstractly, their imagination and fantasy and ability to think out of the box is limited. The reason, according to relevant research, being too much time spent in front of the computer or television. Nerve cell connections in the brain develop differently. Even the active vocabulary is suffering: In the fifties, a 14

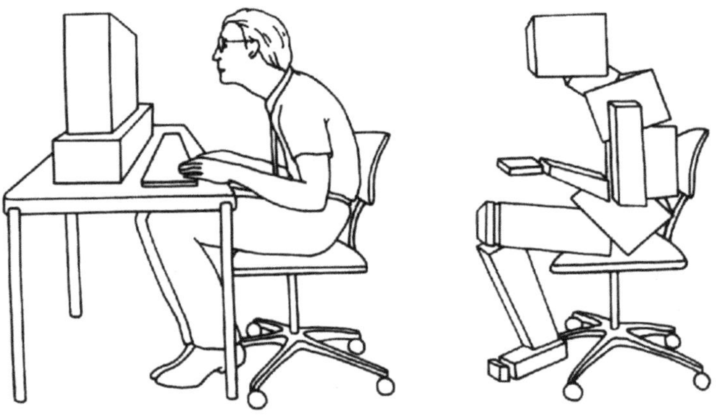

Fig. 34

year old US American boy had an active vocabulary of 25,000 words – today it is 10,000.

Henning Scheich is a German professor for Neurobiology. He postulates that things learnt at school cannot be established in the brain if it is continually superimposed with computer and television images.

In addition, children cannot create any original images or develop their imagination because they are flooded with artificial images.

The study „A Fools Gold: A Critical Look at Computers in Childhood" was published in 2000 in the USA. Repetitive Strain Injury Syndrome occurs above average among children up to the age of 10 who often use the computer. The symptoms are tendonitis and tense muscles which can later make working on a computer impossible. Following the publication of this research, 750 well known researchers demanded a moratorium for the use of computers in early childhood and primary school.

Educationalists like Dr. Bruno Sandkuehler emphasise that the best way to get children away from the screen is strengthening the family through doing things together. And, last but not least, a television should in general not be placed in a childresn´s room.

References:

Susanne Paulsen, Cyberkids – Begegnung mit einer fluechtigen Spezies, in: *Geo Wissen* April 2003

Spiegel 21/2002, p.184

Studie des Kriminologischen Forschungsinstituts Niedersachsen, Hannover 2003

Dr. Bruno Sandkuehler (Pedagoge and member of the European Council), 2004

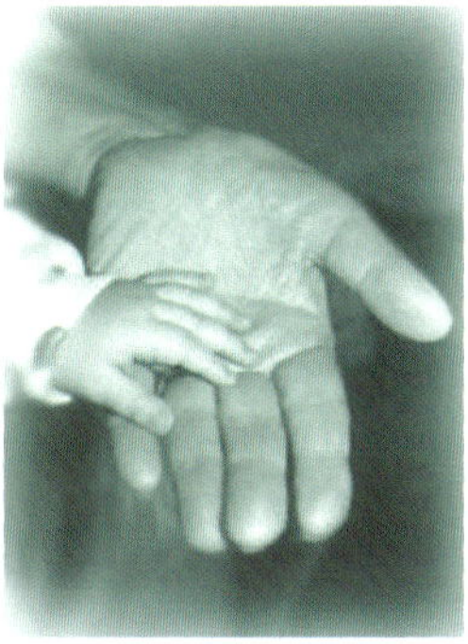

Addresses and Literature

1. Addresses

You can ask for a list of Rolfers (SI-practitioners being educated by the Rolf Institute) in your area at the following address:

* **Rolf Institute® of Structural Integration**
  5055 Chaparral Court
  Boulder, CO 80301 (USA)
  Phone: 303-449-5903
  info@rol.org
  www.rolf.org

A list of Structural Integration practitioners of various schools of SI is available from:

* **International Association of Structural Integrators (IASI)**
  7044 S. 13th Street
  Oak Creek, WI 53154 (USA)
  Phone: 414-908-4947
  Info@TheIASI.org
  www.theiasi.org

2. Literature

- *Ida P. Rolf,* Rolfing and Physical Reality, Healing Arts Press 1990
- *Ida P. Rolf,* Rolfing: Reestablishing the Natural Alignment and Structural Integration of the Human Body for Vitality and Well-Being, Healing Arts Press 1989
- *Hans Georg Brecklinghaus*, Rolfing – Structural Integration. What it achieves, how it works and whom it helps, Lebenshaus Verlag 2004
- *Michaele Glockner,* A Guide to Child Health, Floris Books 2007
- *Magda Gerber,* Dear Parent: Caring for Infants With Respect, Resources for Infant Educators 2003
- *Robert Toporek,* New Book Of Baby And Child Massage, Running Press 2001
- *Peter A. Levine*: Trauma-Proofing Your Kids: A Parents' Guide for Instilling Confidence, Joy and Resilience, North Atlantic Books 2008
- *Ashley Montague,* The Human Significance of the Skin, Harper Paperbacks 1986
- *Richard N. Firshein*, Reversing Asthma, Warner Books 1996

About the Author

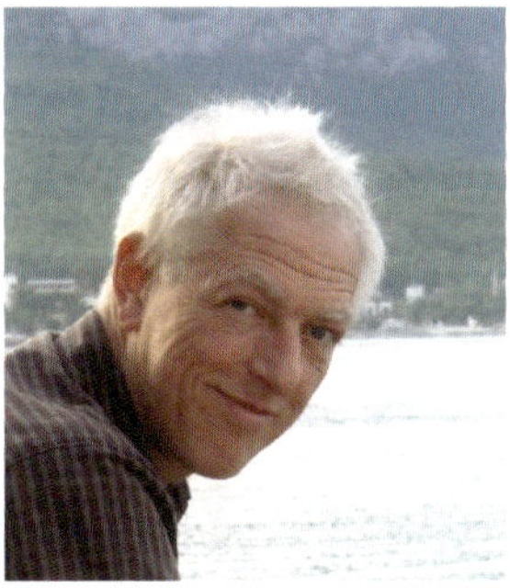

Hans Georg Brecklinghaus has a Degree in Education (Dipl.Paed.), was born 1951 and is a Certified Advanced Rolfer™ and Rolf Movement™ Teacher. He has been practising Rolfing® - Structural Integration in his private practice for 30 years.

Additional qualifications: craniosacral therapy, visceral manipulation and further training in Somatic Experiencing (Trauma Work according to Dr. Peter Levine).

He has many years of work experience as a teacher of *Deutsche Gesellschaft für Strukturelle Integration (DGSI)*. In addition, he is the author of various articles which have been published in specialist literature and of the book: *Rolfing – Structural Integration. What it achieves, how it works and whom it helps*

Address:

Stadtstrasse 9a
D - 79104 Freiburg
Germany
Tel. 0049/+761/42793
hgbreck@online.de
www.rolfing-praxis.de

Illustration References

Hans Georg Brecklinghaus: Fig. 3, 7, 8, 9, 10, 13, 14, 15, 16, 20, 24, 25, 26, 27, 28, 29, 30, 33, illustrations on p.31 and p.117

Hans Flury: Fig. 4, 31, 32

Carlos Repetto: illustration on p.5

Deutsche Gesellschaft für Strukturelle Integration: illustration on p.7

Rolf Institute of Structural Integration: Illustration on front cover and photo on back cover, Fig.1

Unknown: Fig. 2, 5, 6, 11, 12, 17, 18, 19, 21, 22, 23, 34, illustration on p.103, photos on front cover

Available from the same author:

Hans Georg Brecklinghaus

Rolfing-
Structural Integration

What it achieves, how it works and whom it helps

119 pages, 18 Fig., 10,40 $ / 11,95 £
ISBN 978-3-932803-03-5

Lebenshaus Verlag

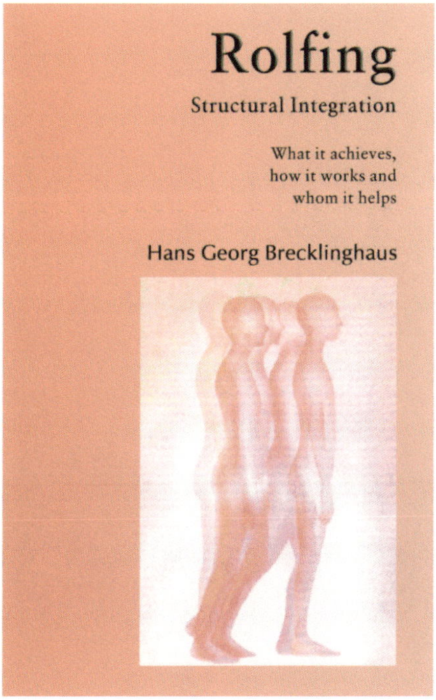

Hans Georg Brecklinghaus

The Human Beings are awoken, You have set them upright

Body Structure and Conception of Man in Ancient Egyptian Art and the Present Day

344 pages, 109 Fig., 28,95 $ / 19,- £

ISBN 978-3-932803-04-3

Lebenshaus Verlag

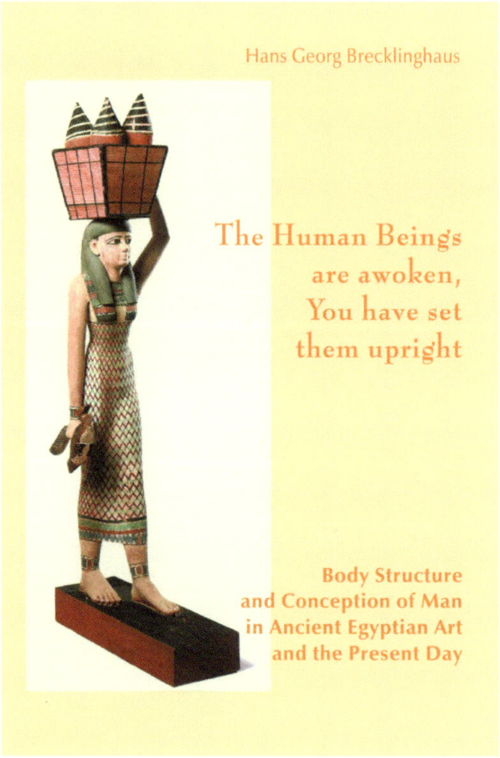

CPSIA information can be obtained at www.ICGtesting.com
Printed in the USA
BVIW12n1440280615
405895BV00020B/6

* 9 7 8 3 9 3 2 8 0 3 1 3 0 *